The Calorie Guide to Branded Foods

D1589699

The Calorie Guide to Branded Foods

by ALEXANDRA SHERMAN

Arlington Books
King Street, St. James's
London

THE CALORIE GUIDE TO
BRANDED FOODS

revised edition July 1984
second impression November 1984
third impression December 1985
fourth impression April 1987
revised edition March 1988

Typeset by Inforum Ltd, Portsmouth
Printed and bound by
The Bath Press, Bath

ISBN 85140 733 1

Acknowledgements

The author is grateful for the co-operation of almost all the companies approached for this the third edition of *The Pocket Calorie Guide to Branded Foods*. It is really remarkable how extremely helpful the people approached have been, once again.

We are delighted to be able to include such companies as *Sainsbury*, *Bejam*, *Holland and Barrett*, *Boots*, together with many smaller manufacturers whose products are widely obtainable.

Our thanks to everyone included in this book.

Contents

Foreword to Third Edition

Those of you who are already in possession of the first or second edition of this pocket book will notice immediately that this third edition is much thicker. This fact means that it has been possible to include many more products, partly because there are so many more available, particularly in the 'main meals' section. Another reason is the huge increase in the number of 'own-name' products from the big supermarket chains.

Those of you who have never seen *The Pocket Calorie Guide to Branded Foods* before should read the foreword to the first edition on page 5 which explains how it can help those people who wish to lose weight (or maintain their weight) without resorting to special 'slimming' foods. The idea is that you are able to eat anything, anywhere although unfortunately *not* in any quantity! With this book in your pocket or bag this should be possible.

Many interesting facts emerge from careful study of the figures in this book, one of which is that — sadly — if something is good for you it does not follow that it is low in calories. Nevertheless you should always try to choose something which is nutritionally good for you when you feel like indulging in those several hundred unnecessary calories! In this edition there are many more of what have come to be known as 'health foods' due to the quantities of new products which have become available during the last 4 years.

The Baked Goods section posed a bit of a problem. Bread does not really belong in a guide to 'branded' foods as calorific content does not vary from brand to brand. However there are many other baked goods available which seemed to fit equally well in either 'bread, buns . . .' or 'cakes, pies . . .' We are sorry, but you may find it necessary to search in both sections to find the product you are looking for.

This book is as comprehensive as is possible but unfortunately the delay between obtaining the figures and actual publication of the book makes it certain that you will not find every possible product included.

Foreword

This little book is aimed primarily at those people—and there are many of us—who always have had and probably always will have what is euphemistically called a 'weight problem'. There are—alas—very few people who can eat whatever they want, in any quantity, without putting on weight. The idea behind this book is that, when used in conjunction with *The Pocket Calorie Guide to Safe Slimming* by Jane Colin, you can eat what you like but easily regulate the quantity to ensure that no weight is gained. It will also, of course, be invaluable to those who have a great deal of weight to lose—nothing is more boring than weeks on end eating only cottage cheese and grapefruit! With this book to help you, there is no reason why you shouldn't have, for example, a piece of cake for tea, as long as it is carefully weighed and the calories included with your allowance for the day. In this book you will be able to find the actual brand name of the piece of cake you wish to eat, so no mistakes need be made; after all, 'one medium slice of chocolate cake' could mean different things to different people. That is why—where possible—weights have been given per ounce and per hundred grammes, so that everything can be properly weighed and there is no excuse for cheating. One exception is biscuits, since most of the manufacturers in this category supplied only the figures per biscuit, and it was therefore necessary to list them in this way.

It must be stressed that before embarking on any diet you should confirm with your doctor that you are in good health. For somebody who is very overweight it can be a considerable shock to the system to reduce the calorie intake drastically, so please tell your doctor what you are planning to do. In most cases doctors will approve wholeheartedly. At this point I should add that, although the figures quoted are quite accurate enough for a weight loss diet, they should not be used by anybody who must limit or avoid any particular food-stuff for medical reasons.

It is advisable to go out and buy a good, accurate pair of scales. I find the type used for mail to be extremely useful. It can be all too easy to cheat using ordinary kitchen scales!

So, you have this book, and probably another book which lists the calorie content of foods in their natural state, and you are all set to get your weight down to its correct level (there is a table at the end of the Foreword giving average weights for men and women). To do this, you must find out by trial and error to what level you, personally, must reduce your intake of calories in order to achieve your required weight loss per week (always think in terms of per week, and not per day, as it can be very depressing to weigh yourself daily since you cannot expect to lose every day). This level should never go below 750 calories per day if you are leading a normal life. It is fine to starve yourself for a couple of days if you are able to relax and do nothing—but this is not the way to achieve a permanent weight loss. In any case this particular book is certainly not for those who wish to starve themselves, but rather for those who want to be able to eat what they enjoy, and enjoy what they eat!

Most *average* people will achieve a satisfactory weight loss (I must stress *average*, as each body is different) on 1000 calories per day for women, and 1200–1500 per day for men. But even on 500 more that that per day respectively, you will still lose weight, albeit slowly. Once your desired weight is reached, in order to avoid gaining weight a satisfactory daily allowance is 2250 calories for most women, and slightly more for most men. But, and this cannot be repeated too often, each person is different, and to begin with it has to be a case of trial and error. If you find you are gaining weight on 2250 calories per day then you must reduce the daily allowance and try again.

This little calorie guide can be used by anybody —either to lose weight, or, once this has been achieved, to maintain the ideal figure. The causes and effects of obesity are gone into in greater detail in Jane Colin's *New Pocket Calorie Guide to Safe Slimming*, but there is only one possible cure—*eat less*. With this book this should be fairly easy without too much suffering. Good luck!

You may wonder why no so-called 'slimming foods' have been included in this book. This was a calculated decision. The nutritional content (including calories) of all such foods is carefully listed on the packaging and, as we want to keep this *pocket* book as concise as possible, we feel it to be unnecessary to include them.

The figures given have been supplied by the manufacturers very recently but, unfortunately, it may be that by the time the book is published some of the products will have been discontinued and other new ones will have appeared. This is unavoidable, and the tables will be updated as often as possible for each new edition. It is also impossible to list every food-stuff available in Britain, but if you find a particular brand-name food missing you will probably be able to find an equivalent under a different name. Although this is by no means ideal, it is better to use the figures from another brand-name than not to count the calories at all!

WHAT YOU SHOULD WEIGH

The following weight table is of necessity only average. Each person has an ideal weight at which they look and feel their best. A person with large bones can weigh as much as half a stone more than somebody with small bones and still look very good. The best way to find out whether you are large, medium or small boned is to measure your wrist (and no cheating!).

For women: wrists measuring 5½" mean small bones; 6–6½" mean medium bones; over 6½" mean large bones.

For men: wrists measuring 6½"–7" mean small bones; 7"–7½" mean medium bones; over 8" mean large bones.

So use the following tables only as a guideline. Those of you with small or large bones should deduct or add between five and seven pounds (two to three kilos) from these weights.

AVERAGE WEIGHTS TABLE

(These weights include no clothes. For light clothing but no shoes you should add three pounds (1.4 kilos)).

MEN				WOMEN			
Height Ft. Ins.	St.	Weight Lbs.	Kilos	Height Ft. Ins.	St.	Weight Lbs.	Kilos
5 0	8	10	55.5	4 8	7	8	48.2
5 1	8	12	56.4	4 9	7	10	49.1
5 2	9	0	57.3	4 10	7	12	50.0
5 3	9	3	58.6	4 11	8	0	50.9
5 4	9	6	60.0	5 0	8	2	51.8
5 5	9	10	61.8	5 1	8	4	52.7
5 6	10	0	63.6	5 2	8	6	53.6
5 7	10	4	65.5	5 3	8	11	55.9
5 8	10	8	67.3	5 4	8	13	56.8
5 9	10	12	69.1	5 5	9	2	58.2
5 10	11	3	71.4	5 6	9	6	60.0
5 11	11	8	73.6	5 7	9	10	61.8
6 0	12	0	76.4	5 8	10	0	63.6
6 1	12	6	79.1	5 9	10	4	65.5
6 2	12	12	81.8	5 10	10	8	67.3
6 3	13	4	84.5	5 11	10	11	68.6
6 4	13	10	87.3	6 0	11	1	70.5

Biscuits — Sweet

Biscuits are definitely not a recommended foodstuff for anybody on a serious slimming diet. However, if you can restrict yourself to one or two they are a pleasant treat every now and again. The problem is, of course, not to eat an entire packet!

Food	Quantities	Calories	Quantities	Calories
ALLINSON				
Bran	1 biscuit	53	100 g	421
'Carob Coated'				
Carob Bites	"	25	"	480
Fruit & Nut	"	84	"	505
Ginger & Bran	"	73	"	438
Oatmeal	"	81	"	483
Raisin & Bran	"	86	"	514
Coconut & Nutmeg	"	63	"	464
Fruit & Nut	"	56	"	410
Ginger	"	57	"	430
Hazelnut	"	62	"	458
Honey	"	55	"	402
Muesli	"	61	"	450
Oatmeal	"	59	"	431

Biscuits — Sweet

Food	Quantities	Calories	Quantities	Calories
Scottish Shortbread	1 biscuit	82	100 g	494
Soft Bake Coconut Cookies	2 biscuits	115	"	458
Soft Bake Raisin & Bran	"	94	"	377
BOOTS				
Coconut & Honey	1 oz	154	100 g	541
Fig & Orange	"	137	"	484
Ginger & Lemon	"	146	"	514
Sultana & Bran	"	138	"	485
'Second Nature'				
Apple	"	126	"	443
Bran	"	123	"	433
Fruit/Bran	"	119	"	418
Hazelnut	"	127	"	448
Honey	"	125	"	441
Muesli/Fruit	"	131	"	461
Shortbread	"	135	"	476
Six Grain	"	125	"	441
CADBURY				
Animals	1 biscuit	30	100 g	480
Bournville Assorted	"	60	"	500
Bournville Digestives	"	45	"	480
Butter Shorties	"	45	"	475
Chocolate Cabarets	"	45	"	470
Chocolate & Orange	"	60	"	470
Coconut Coasters	"	45	"	485
Fingers	"	25	"	495

Food	Quantities	Calories	Quantities	Calories
Fruit & Nut Cookes	1 biscuit	45	100 g	450
Ginger & Hazelnut	"	65	"	485
Honey & Almond	"	60	"	470
Milk Assorted	"	60	"	495
Milk Digestive	"	50	"	490
Orange Cremes	"	80	"	500
Original Cookies	"	50	"	490

CRAWFORD

Food	Quantities	Calories
Balmoral Fingers	1 biscuit	65
'Cookie Bags'	"	39
Choc Chip & Caramel	"	39
Choc Chip & Hazelnut	"	39
Choc Chip & Orange	"	39
Marie	"	33
Mini Cookies	"	16
'Pennywise'		
Bourbon Creams	"	62
Coconut Creams	"	67
Custard Creams	"	66
Fig Rolls	"	57
Finger Nice	"	26
Frosted Creams	"	43
Garibaldi	"	46
Iced Shorties	"	42
Jam Rings	"	61
Malties	"	36
Morning Coffee	"	21

Biscuits — Sweet

Food	Quantities	Calories	Quantities	Calories
Orange Cream	1 biscuit	63		
Raspberry Cream	"	66		
Shortcake	"	53		
Shorties	"	37		
Tea Fingers	"	22		
Wafer	"	47		
Thin Arrowroot	"	30		
'Shortbread'				
Highland Fingers	"	63		
Petticoat Tails	"	57		
Tartan Shortbread	"	97		
DOVE'S FARM				
Bourbon	1 biscuit	60	100 g	477
Carob Coated Digestives	"	63	"	499
Digestive	"	56	"	470
Ginger Nuts	"	32	"	432
FORTTS				
Bath Oliver	1 biscuit	45	100 g	375
Chocolate Bath Oliver	"	88	"	359
HOLLY MILLS				
Carob Chip	1 biscuit	60	100 g	444
Farmhouse	"	49	"	437
Fig & Oat	"	65	"	384

Food	Quantities	Calories	Quantities	Calories
Fruit & Nut	1 biscuit	66	100 g	403
Ginger	,,	57	,,	439
Lemon Crunch	,,	58	,,	450
Peanut & Sesame	,,	56	,,	447
'Slym-Range'				
Shortcake	,,	33	,,	438
Slymbran Digestives	,,	37	,,	443
Slymsquares	,,	30	,,	497
'Snack Packs'				
Ginger Crunch	,,	57	,,	439
Lemon Crunch	,,	58	,,	450
Oat and Honey Crunch	,,	49	,,	437
HUNTLEY & PALMER				
Butter Biscuit	1 biscuit	48	100 g	469
Cherry Sultana	,,	N/A	,,	304
Chop Chip 'N' Nut Cookie	,,	45	,,	488
Coconut Biscuit	,,	51	,,	511
Digestive	,,	63	,,	463
Digestive, chocolate	,,	65	,,	502
Digestive, Fruit	,,	50	,,	451
Dutch shortcake	,,	40	,,	539
Lemon Puff	,,	80	,,	521
Raisin Biscuit	,,	59	,,	454
Sponge Finger	,,	21	,,	388
Syrup (Kennett)	,,	63	,,	500

Biscuits — Sweet

Food	Quantities	Calories	Quantities	Calories
JACOB				
'Club'				
Coffee	1 biscuit	113	100 g	503
Fruit	"	113	"	471
Milk	"	117	"	410
Orange	"	113	"	497
Plain	"	112	"	494
Mint	"	113	"	495
Wafer	"	100	"	517
Farmhouse	"	39	"	488
Fig Roll	"	54	"	355
Trio	"	127	"	530
MCDONALD'S				
Taxi	1 biscuit	81		
Yoyo Mint	"	100		
Yoyo Toffee	"	98		
MCVITIE'S				
Abbey Crunch	1 biscuit	47		
Abbey Crunch Cream	"	69		
Bandit	"	105		
'Country Cookies'				
Almond & Honey	"	86		
Cherry & Coconut	"	84		
Digestive	"	74		
Digestive Cream	"	69		

Food	Quantities	Calories	Quantities	Calories
Finger, Milk & Plain				
chocolate	1 biscuit	25		
54321	"	100		
Fruit Shortcake	"	50		
Gingernut	"	46		
Gipsy Cream	"	69		
Hobnob	"	71		
milk chocolate	"	80		
plain chocolate	"	80		
Homewheat				
milk chocolate	"	84		
plain chocolate	"	85		
Jaffa Cake	"	48		
Lincoln	"	48		
Munchmallow	"	81		
Mickey	"	107		
'Natural Choice'				
Blackcurrant Yoghurt				
Cream	"	69		
Fruit & Nut Crunch	"	49		
Muesli Cookie	"	86		
Wholemeal	"	61		
Yoghurt Cream	"	69		
Penguin	"	125		
Rich Tea	"	35		
Solar Choc Chip	"	110		
Solar Tropical Fruit	"	97		

Biscuits — Sweet

Food	Quantities	Calories	Quantities	Calories
Sports	1 biscuit	107		
United Extra Time	"	223		
United Orange	"	110		
MARKS & SPENCER				
'Assortments'				
All Butter Shortbread	1 oz	145	100 g	510
Fancy Biscuits	"	125	"	439
Speciality	"	143	"	504
'Chocolate'				
Break In	"	168	"	590
Chocolate Cream Tartlets	"	125	"	440
Crunchy Sandwich Bar	"	142	"	499
Florentines	"	155	"	545
Jaffa Cakes	"	105	"	369
Milk Chocolate				
Caramel Wafer	"	129	"	455
Crunch	"	137	"	483
Currant Topped				
Caramel Wafer	"	137	"	481
Digestive	"	142	"	500
Fruit & Nut Cereal Bar	"	140	"	494
Malted Milk Chocolate				
Sandwich Bar	"	149	"	526
Orange Sandwich	"	148	"	522
Sandwich	"	144	"	507
Teacake	"	125	"	440

Food	Quantities	Calories	Quantities	Calories
Plain Chocolate				
Biscuit Thin	1 oz	140	100 g	494
Digestive	”	143	”	505
Ginger Biscuit	”	139	”	490
Mint Sandwich Bar	”	139	”	491
'Cookies'				
All Butter Sultana	”	125	”	442
Chocolate Chip				
& Hazelnut	”	143	”	502
Chocolate Chip	”	140	”	494
Muesli	”	135	”	476
Viennese Chocolate				
Sandwich	”	145	”	510
'Cream Biscuits'				
Bourbon	”	138	”	487
Butter Crunch	”	143	”	503
Fruit & Nut	”	131	”	460
Rich Tea Finger	”	136	”	479
'Speciality Biscuits'				
Apple Crumble				
Cookies	”	124	”	437
Black Cherry Tartlet	”	110	”	386
Break	”	143	”	502
Luxury Petits Fours	”	146	”	515
Milk Choc. Peanut				
Crunch Bar	”	145	”	509
Meringue Nest	”	109	”	380

Biscuits — Sweet

Food	Quantities	Calories	Quantities	Calories
Milk Chocolate Finger Wafer	1 oz	147	100 g	518
Milk Chocolate Toffee Cup	"	139	"	490
Rainbow Bright	"	145	"	511
Strawberry Tartlet	"	110	"	386
'Standard Biscuits'				
All Butter	"	136	"	481
All Butter Shortbread Finger	"	149	"	525
All Butter Thistle Shortbread	"	146	"	515
Almond	"	144	"	506
Butter Crunch	"	131	"	463
Digestive	"	141	"	499
Fruit & Nut Cereal Bar	"	126	"	444
Fruit Shortcake	"	135	"	476
Ginger Snap	"	120	"	423
Malted Milk	"	132	"	466
Rich Tea	"	131	"	460
Rich Tea Finger	"	130	"	459
Round Shorties	"	140	"	494
Wheaten Sweetmeal	"	129	"	453
PEAK FREAN				
Bourbon	1 biscuit	60	100 g	468
Chocolate Triple	"	180	"	541
Citrus Cream	"	58	"	480

Food	Quantities	Calories	Quantities	Calories
Coated Mallow Milk/Orange	1 biscuit	52	100 g	433
Coconut Mallow	,,	46	,,	384
Coffee Cream	,,	56	,,	480
Country Crunch	,,	36	,,	445
Crunch Cream	,,	58	,,	482
Currant Crisp	,,	30	,,	440
Custard Cream	,,	53	,,	483
Devon Cream	,,	58	,,	487
Digestive, small	,,	48	,,	490
Fruit Shortcake	,,	36	,,	443
Garibaldi	,,	32	,,	358
Ginger Nut	,,	36	,,	431
Iced Gem	,,	5	,,	380
Jaffa Crunch	,,	30	,,	444
Jamboree Mallow	,,	77	,,	382
Jersey Cream	,,	58	,,	482
Lincoln	,,	35	,,	486
Malt Crunch	,,	35	,,	420
Megabar	,,	97	,,	376
Neapolitan Wafer	,,	36	,,	504
Nice	,,	44	,,	449
Nice Cream	,,	57	,,	484
Orange Cream	,,	57	,,	473
Rich Osborne	,,	35	,,	437
Rich Tea	,,	25	,,	438
Shortcake	,,	49	,,	454

Biscuits — Sweet

Food	Quantities	Calories	Quantities	Calories
Snow Ball	1 biscuit	131	100 g	418
Treacle Crunch	"	29	"	436
SAFEWAY				
All Butter	1 oz	137	100 g	481
All Butter Fruit	"	135	"	475
Almond	"	144	"	506
Bourbon Cream	"	127	"	446
Butter Crinkle	"	127	"	449
Butter Shorties	"	138	"	487
Butter Crunch Cream	"	141	"	498
Chocolate Cream	"	138	"	485
Choc Nut Cookie	"	141	"	495
Coconut Sandwich Cream	"	133	"	470
Coconut Ring	"	128	"	451
Cornish Cream	"	143	"	502
Currant Crunch	"	128	"	450
Custard Cream	"	144	"	507
Digestive	"	136	"	480
Fig Roll	"	96	"	340
Finger Cream	"	136	"	478
Fruit Shortcake	"	135	"	477
Ginger Cream	"	139	"	488
Ginger Nut	"	121	"	426
Golden Crunch Cream	"	144	"	506
Iced Ring	"	126	"	443
Jam Sandwich Cream	"	133	"	470

Food	Quantities	Calories	Quantities	Calories
Lemon Cream	1 oz	136	100 g	478
Lemon Puff	"	148	"	521
Milk Chocolate				
Caramel Wafer	"	161	"	567
Caramel Shortcake	"	136	"	478
Finger	"	150	"	528
Digestive Bar	"	145	"	510
Fruit & Nut Bar	"	141	"	498
Orange Finger	"	138	"	487
Orange Sandwich	"	144	"	506
Sandwich	"	144	"	506
Sunota	"	142	"	500
Shortcake	"	146	"	516
Nice Finger	"	136	"	478
Oaten Crunch	"	130	"	459
Plain Chocolate				
Crunch	"	136	"	478
Digestive	"	142	"	500
Finger	"	160	"	562
Petticoat Tail	"	132	"	465
Rich Tea	"	128	"	451
Rydal	"	135	"	475
Shortbread Finger	"	131	"	461
Shortcake	"	143	"	502
Shorties	"	140	"	495
Snowball	"	71	"	251
Sport	"	134	"	473

Biscuits — Sweet

Food	Quantities	Calories	Quantities	Calories
Wafer	1 oz	134	100 g	473
Cream	,,	143	,,	505
SAINSBURY				
All Butter Crunch	1 biscuit	34		
Assorted	,,	55		
Bourbon	,,	65		
Butter Sandwich Cream	1 oz	143	100 g	505
Caramel Wafer	1 biscuit	85		
Choc-chip Nibble Cookies	,,	15		
Choc-chip Shortbread Ring	,,	65		
Chocolate Malted Milk	,,	45		
Chocolate and Nut Cookie	,,	45		
Chocolate Sandwich Wafer	,,	90		
Chocolate Tea Cake	,,	70		
Coconut Cookie	,,	45		
Crunch Cream	,,	70		
Custard Cream	,,	55		
Fig Roll	,,	30		
Fruit Digestive	,,	50		
Fruit & Nut Cream	,,	60		
Fruit Shortcake	,,	35		
Garibaldi	,,	30		
Ginger Cream	,,	70		
Ginger Snap	,,	35		
Iced Bears	,,	37		
Honey & Bran Crunch	,,	45		

Food	Quantities	Calories	Quantities	Calories
Jaffa Cake	1 biscuit	42		
Lemon Crisp	,,	40		
Lemon Puff	,,	75		
Lincoln	,,	45		
Mallow	,,	45		
Malted Milk	,,	35		
Marie	,,	30		
Milk Chocolate Digestive	,,	65		
Milk Chocolate Finger	,,	24		
Morning Coffee	,,	20		
Nice	,,	42		
Oatmeal Crunch	,,	30		
Peanut Crunch	,,	45		
Petticoat Tail Shortbread	,,	50		
Plain Chocolate Digestive	,,	65		
Rich Tea	,,	35		
Sandwich Cream	,,	90		
Shortbread Finger	,,	90		
Shortcake	,,	35		
Shortie	,,	45		
Spicy Fruit Crunch	,,	45		
Snowball	,,	105		
Sponge Finger	,,	18		
Thistle Shortbread	,,	105		
Treacle Crunch Cream	1 oz	126	100 g	445
Wholemeal Honey Sandwich	1 biscuit	75		
Wholemeal Shortbread	,,	75		

Biscuits — Sweet

Food	Quantities	Calories	Quantities	Calories
SPAR				
Bourbon Cream	1 oz	139	100 g	486
Choc'n'Nut Cookie	"	140	"	494
Chocolate Chip Cookie	"	138	"	485
Chocolate Mallow	"	127	"	446
Coconut Crumble Cream	"	148	"	521
Custard Cream	"	144	"	507
Digestive Sweetmeal	"	141	"	493
Fig Roll	"	99	"	350
Fruit Shortcake	"	134	"	471
Ginger Nut	"	140	"	426
Jaffa Cake	"	111	"	390
Jam Ring	"	131	"	462
Milk Chocolate				
Digestive	"	145	"	510
Sandwich	"	144	"	506
Sweetmeal	"	142	"	499
Morning Coffee	"	130	"	458
Nice	"	143	"	505
Orange Cream	"	143	"	505
Plain Chocolate Sweetmeal	"	143	"	505
Rich Tea	"	131	"	460
Rich Tea Finger	"	130	"	459
Shortbread Finger	"	148	"	520
Shortcake	"	145	"	509
Shorties	"	141	"	495

Food	Quantities	Calories	Quantities	Calories
WAITROSE				
Almond	1 oz	145	100 g	510
Butter	,,	136	,,	480
Butter Crunch	,,	129	,,	456
Cafe Noir	,,	111	,,	391
Chocolate Chip	,,	149	,,	524
Chocolate & Nut	,,	142	,,	510
'Chocolate Coated'				
Almond Crunch, Milk	,,	144	,,	507
Breaktime				
Milk	,,	168	,,	590
Plain	,,	167	,,	588
Crisp Caramel Wafer, Milk	,,	143	,,	502
Digestive				
Milk	,,	142	,,	499
Plain	,,	143	,,	505
Ginger Crunch Bar, Plain	,,	142	,,	499
Ginger Crunch Biscuit	,,	134	,,	472
Chocolate Mint Sandwich,				
Plain	,,	147	,,	519
Muesli Crunch Bar				
Milk	,,	141	,,	496
Plain	,,	140	,,	495
Orange Sandwich	,,	147	,,	517
Orange Wafer, Milk	,,	133	,,	470
Petit Beurre				
Milk	,,	133	,,	470

Biscuits — Sweet

Food	Quantities	Calories	Quantities	Calories
Plain	1 oz	133	100 g	470
Wafer Finger				
Milk	”	136	”	480
Plain	”	143	”	504
Plain Mint	”	145	”	510
Coconut Cookies	”	139	”	490
Coconut Crumble Cream	”	148	”	521
Coconut Ring	”	139	”	490
Coffee Cream	”	135	”	476
Crunchy Cookies	”	126	”	443
Crunchy Cream	”	144	”	506
Custard Cream	”	144	”	507
Digestive	”	139	”	490
Digestive Finger Cream	”	139	”	489
Fruit Shortcake	”	135	”	476
Garibaldi	”	105	”	370
Ginger Cream	”	139	”	488
Ginger Snap	”	121	”	428
Ginger Thin	”	129	”	456
Hazelnut Cookies	”	140	”	493
Highland Shorties	”	141	”	495
Iced Ring	”	126	”	443
Jam Cream	”	176	”	479
Malted Milk	”	132	”	466
Muesli	”	127	”	448
Nice	”	130	”	457
Oatflake & Honey	”	136	”	479

Biscuits — Sweet

Food	Quantities	Calories	Quantities	Calories
Petit Beurre	1 oz	133	100 g	468
Petticoat Tail	"	145	"	509
Rich Tea	"	131	"	460
Rich Tea Finger	"	130	"	458
Shortbread Finger	"	144	"	507
Sponge Finger	"	123	"	433
Stem Ginger Cookies	"	138	"	487
Treacle Cookies	"	145	"	511
Treacle Crunch Cream	"	141	"	495
Wholemeal Shortbread Finger	"	141	"	495

Biscuits — Savoury

There is such a wide range of delicious products in this category on the market now, imported from all over the world, that it should be possible for you to indulge (prudently) in something really pleasing to the palate without exceeding your daily calorie allowance. For obvious reasons it is better to choose biscuits with a high fibre content, of which there are many available.

Food	Quantities	Calories	Quantities	Calories
ALLINSON				
Bran Oatcake	1 biscuit	51	100 g	419
Wholemeal Crispbread	”	15	”	344
BUITONI				
Grissini	1 oz	102	100 g	360
Melba Toast	”	108	”	382

Food	Quantities	Calories	Quantities	Calories
CARRS				
Table Water				
large	1 biscuit	33		
small	"	15		
CRAWFORDS				
Butter Puff	1 biscuit	50		
Cream Cracker	"	38		
HOLLY MILLS				
'Fibre Time'				
Cheese & Chilli	1 biscuit	25	100 g	451
Cheese & Onion	"	25	"	467
Curry	"	25	"	454
Fibre Time	"	71	"	329
'Slym-Range'				
Original	1 slice	11	100 g	343
Rye	"	12	"	338
Sesame	"	15	"	367
Wholemeal	"	12	"	327
JACOB				
Cornish Wafer	1 biscuit	43	100 g	514
Cream Cracker	"	33	"	431
Rich table Water	"	30	"	411
Table Cracker	"	33	"	431
Thinner Water	"	27	"	387

Biscuits — Savoury

Food	Quantities	Calories	Quantities	Calories
Water	1 biscuit	31	100 g	394
Water, High Bake	"	31	"	394
MCVITIE'S				
Cheddar	1 biscuit	22		
Mini Cheddar	"	8		
Krackawheat	"	36		
Oatcakes	"	45		
Toasted Golden Crisp	"	22		
Toasted Wheat Crisp	"	22		
TUC	"	26		
TUC Savoury Sandwich	"	78		
MARKS & SPENCER				
Bran Sunnywheat Cracker	1 oz	108	100 g	380
Butter Puff	"	144	"	508
Butterfly Cracker	"	137	"	483
Cheese Bite	"	138	"	485
Cheese Sandwich	"	152	"	535
Cheese Snap	"	147	"	517
Cheese Straw	"	141	"	495
Cheese Thin	"	151	"	533
Herb Thin	"	148	"	522
Onion Kite	"	131	"	463
Round High Baked Water	"	110	"	387
Rye Light Crispbread	"	106	"	375
Savoury Cocktail Biscuit	"	163	"	575

Food	Quantities	Calories	Quantities	Calories
Sesame Cracker	1 oz	132	100 g	465
Walnut Thin	"	143	"	504
Wheaten Cracker	"	139	"	488
Wholemeal Bran	"	123	"	433
Wholemeal Cracker	"	129	"	456
NABISCO				
Cheese Sandwich	1 biscuit	48	100 g	528
Cheese & Onion Sandwich	"	47	"	522
Cheese Ritz Cracker	"	16	"	480
Hovis Cracker	"	29	"	468
Hovis Digestive	"	57	"	486
Ritz Cracker	"	16	"	495
Teabreak	"	38	"	420
Wholewheat Teabreak	"	38	"	388
PEAK FREAN				
Cheeselet	1 biscuit	3	100 g	345
Cheese Stick	"	22	"	539
Cheese & Onion Stick	"	22	"	538
Cheese & Tomato Stick	"	22	"	517
Twiglets				
large	"	6	"	400
small	"	2	"	400
SAFEWAY				
Bath Oliver	1 oz	106	100 g	375

Biscuits — Savoury

Food	Quantities	Calories	Quantities	Calories
Cornish Wafer	1 oz	145	100 g	509
Cream Cracker	,,	132	,,	431
Dixie Cracker	,,	122	,,	431
Farmhouse Cracker	,,	145	,,	509
Oyster Cracker	,,	122	,,	431
Ritz Cracker	,,	131	,,	461
Small Digestive	,,	135	,,	477
Small Water	,,	114	,,	402
Table Cracker	,,	122	,,	431
Water Biscuit	,,	110	,,	387
Water High Bake	,,	110	,,	387
Wheat Cracker	,,	125	,,	442
Wholemeal Bran	,,	122	,,	431

Bread, Buns, etc

In this new edition it has been decided to leave this section exactly as it was in the previous one. Certain companies now produce many interesting baked goods suitable as substitutes for bread. These have been included with cakes in the next section. Meanwhile, with all the products listed below it is *most* important to weigh them carefully. A slice of bread weighing 1 oz or 30 g looks remarkably skinny on the plate and a slice cut by you from a freshly baked loaf is much more likely to weigh 100 g!

Food	Quantities	Calories	Quantities	Calories
Bath Buns	1 oz	88	100 g	310
Brown Bread	"	72	"	254
Brown Bread with Bran	"	71	"	250
Crumpets	"	54	"	190
Currant Buns (no butter)	"	90	"	317
Granary Bread	"	64	"	225
'High Protein' Bread	"	71	"	250

Bread, Buns, etc

Food	Quantities	Calories	Quantities	Calories
Malt Loaf	1 oz	85	100 g	300
Scones	"	90	"	317
Scotch Pancakes	"	87	"	307
White Bread	"	73	"	257
100% Wholemeal Bread	"	78	"	274

Cakes, Pies, Cake Mixes, Pastries & Rolls

The products listed in this section should be of no interest to anybody seriously trying to lose weight. The calorific content of almost all of them is so high that they are best avoided. However there will come a time when you have already indulged and will wish to know how many calories to deduct from your daily allowance. For occasions such as these here is a fairly comprehensive list.

Food	Quantities	Calories	Quantities	Calories
BEJAM *(frozen)*				
Choux Pastry	1 oz	95	100 g	334
Cocktail Vol-au-Vents	,,	43	,,	151
Medium Vol-au-Vents	,,	69	,,	243
Puff Pastry	,,	134	,,	472
Shortcrust Pastry	,,	140	,,	493
BIRD'S EYE *(frozen)*				
Pastry	1 oz	120	100 g	422

Cakes, Pies, Cake Mixes, Pastries & Rolls

Food	Quantities	Calories	Quantities	Calories
Puff Pastry Sheets	1 sheet	360		
Shortcrust Pastry	1 oz	125	100 g	440
Vol-au-Vent Cases	one	70		
CADBURY				
Chocolate Cake	1 oz	111	100 g	392
Coconut Treats	”	116	”	407
5-Milk Chocolate Cakes	”	109	”	384
Flake Cakes	”	140	”	492
Fudge Diamonds	”	139	”	420
Jaffa Fingers	”	119	”	420
Jam Mini Rolls	”	108	”	365
Mini Rolls	”	126	”	444
Swiss Gateau	”	103	”	364
Swiss Roll	”	108	”	379
Whirls	”	104	”	365
GRANNY SMITH'S *(mixes)*				
Butterfly Tops Cake	1 oz	122	100 g	432
Cheesecake	”	62	”	220
Chocolate Sandwich Cake	”	120	”	423
Chocolate Sponge	”	113	”	398
Chocolate Tops Cake	”	100	”	354
Country Harvest				
Brown Bread	”	64	”	225
Crumble	”	129	”	454
Custard	”	22	”	79

Cakes, Pies, Cake Mixes, Pastries & Rolls

Food	Quantities	Calories	Quantities	Calories
Doughnut	1 oz	121	100 g	425
Farmhouse Fruitcake	"	110	"	388
Lemon Madeira Cake	"	93	"	326
Lemon Meringue Crunch	"	71	"	252
Lemon Tops Cake	"	101	"	355
Luxury Sponge	"	97	"	342
Pizza Base	"	70	"	248
Savoury Crumble	"	128	"	451
Scone	"	94	"	330
Shortbread	"	138	"	487
Short Pastry	"	141	"	497
Spicy Cake	"	113	"	398
Suet Dumpling & Pudding	"	97	"	341
White Bread	"	70	"	248
Yorkshire Pudding & Pancake	"	76	"	267

GRANOSE

Fruit Bread	1 oz	87	100 g	310
Wholemeal Toasties	"	115	"	407

JUS-ROL *(frozen)*

Puff Pastry	1 oz	112	100 g	393
Vol-au-Vents	"	112	"	393

LYONS

Apple Almond Slice	1 oz	119	100 g	420

Cakes, Pies, Cake Mixes, Pastries & Rolls

Food	Quantities	Calories	Quantities	Calories
Bakewell Tarts	1 oz	100 g	420	
Battenberg	"	102	"	358
Blackcurrant Puffs	"	129	"	453
Butter Madeira	"	107	"	378
Chocolate Fancies	"	127	"	449
Chocolate and Caramel Rolls	"	124	"	437
Chocolate and Jam Rolls	"	109	"	385
Chocolate Sandwich	"	107	"	378
Coconut & Apricot Slice	"	129	"	454
Cup Cakes				
Chocolate	"	96	"	338
Orange/Lemon	"	102	"	361
Date & Apple Slices	"	105	"	371
Fingers				
Chocolate	"	118	"	414
Strawberry	"	104	"	368
Flan	"	91	"	320
French Sandwich	"	104	"	369
Fruit Pies				
Apple	"	107	"	376
Apple & Blackcurrant	"	110	"	387
Harvest	"	109	"	384
Fruit & Syrup Cake	"	114	"	401
Lemon Meringues	"	108	"	382
Madeleines				
Apricot	"	96	"	335
Raspberry	"	95	"	333

Food	Quantities	Calories	Quantities	Calories
Paradise Slices	1 oz	121	100 g	426
Pies				
Apple dessert	”	99	”	349
Apple Popular	”	99	”	349
Apple & Blackcurrant				
Popular	”	100	”	353
Apricot Popular	”	100	”	353
Blackcurrant & Apple				
Lattice	”	92	”	324
Cherry Apple Lattice	”	89	”	314
Sponge Sandwich, Raspberry	”	89	”	314
Sundaes				
Apricot	”	112	”	396
Blackcurrant & Apple	”	110	”	389
Swiss Roll				
Chocolate/Vanilla	”	106	”	373
Raspberry	”	85	”	298
Raspberry & Vanilla	”	96	”	340
Tarts				
Iced	”	118	”	417
Jam	”	118	”	414
Trifle Sponge	”	87	”	308
Viennese Whirls	”	146	”	516
MARKS & SPENCER *(large cakes)*				
All Butter Madeira Cut	1 oz	114	100 g	401

Cakes, Pies, Cake Mixes, Pastries & Rolls

Food	Quantities	Calories	Quantities	Calories
Angel Sandwich	1 oz	163	100 g	574
Apricot Sponge Roll	ʺ	100	ʺ	352
Apple Sponge Sandwich	ʺ	68	ʺ	240
Banana Madeira Sandwich	ʺ	110	ʺ	389
Battenburg	ʺ	102	ʺ	361
Butter Walnut Sandwich	ʺ	117	ʺ	412
Caramel	ʺ	121	ʺ	425
Carrot	ʺ	101	ʺ	357
Cheesecake, Baked Lemon	ʺ	70	ʺ	248
Cherry Madeira Cut Cake	ʺ	114	ʺ	403
Chocolate Sponge Roll with Chocolate Buttercream	ʺ	114	ʺ	403
Coconut Cake	ʺ	118	ʺ	415
Country Cake	ʺ	121	ʺ	428
Jam Swiss Roll	ʺ	89	ʺ	312
Parkin Cut Cake	ʺ	93	ʺ	329
Raspberry Sponge Sandwich with fresh cream	ʺ	85	ʺ	300
Sponge Gateau				
Buttercream/Jam	ʺ	111	ʺ	391
Chocolate B/Cream	ʺ	117	ʺ	413
Sponge Sandwich –				
Buttercream/Jam	ʺ	120	ʺ	424
Sultana & Cherry Cake	ʺ	77	ʺ	273
Walnut Sponge Roll	ʺ	119	ʺ	418
(frozen)				
Chocolate Layer Cake	ʺ	96	ʺ	340

Cakes, Pies, Cake Mixes, Pastries & Rolls

Food	Quantities	Calories	Quantities	Calories
Strawberry Cream Gateau	1 oz	64	100 g	225
(Christmas lines)				
All Butter Rich Fruit	"	106	"	368
with Iced Top	"	97	"	342
with Marzipan	"	104	"	368
with Marzipan & Icing	"	96	"	337
Cherry Genoa –				
square, decorated	"	95	"	334
Chocolate Christmas Log	"	118	"	415
(small cakes)				
Black Forest Gateau Slices	"	91	"	320
Chocolate Covered				
Mini Rolls	"	122	"	430
Chocolate Eclairs	"	117	"	413
Chocolate Fudge Brownies	"	125	"	441
Chocolate Hexagons	"	125	"	441
Chorley Cakes	"	116	"	408
Choux Buns	"	94	"	330
Corn Crisp	"	138	"	487
Cream Scones	"	96	"	340
Fondant Fancies	"	96	"	339
Fresh Cream Meringues	"	96	"	338
Frozen Cream Doughnuts	"	104	"	365
Rice Crisp with Raisins	"	127	"	448
Rolls, etc				
Aberdeen Rolls	"	120	"	423
Bath Buns	"	119	"	420

Cakes, Pies, Cake Mixes, Pastries & Rolls

Food	Quantities	Calories	Quantities	Calories
Big Country Brown Rolls	1 oz	74	100 g	262
Big Country Rolls – Sesame	”	77	”	270
Breakfast/Morning Rolls	”	72	”	255
Croissants	”	109	”	383
Crusty Cob Rolls	”	80	”	282
Farmhouse Baps	”	76	”	268
Fruited Lardy Cake	”	119	”	419
Fruited Treacle Crumpets	”	79	”	280
Malt Loaf	”	76	”	267
Mini Hovis Loaves	”	71	”	250
Old English & Scottish Rolls	”	79	”	280
Potato Scones	”	60	”	210
Rich Fruit Loaf	”	70	”	245
Scotch Pancakes	”	87	”	305
Sultana & Syrup Pancakes	”	79	”	280
Teacakes	”	77	”	270
MCVITIE'S				
Banana	1 oz	109	100 g	383
Cherry Fruit Pieces	”	93	”	329
Cherry Fruit Slab	”	149	”	524
Cherry Sultana No.2	”	95	”	335
Chocolate Cake	”	40	”	142
Dark Orange	”	38	”	135
Fruit Cake Slice (individually wrapped)	1 slice	148		
Genoa Fruit Pieces	1 oz	98	100 g	347

Cakes, Pies, Cake Mixes, Pastries & Rolls

Food	Quantities	Calories	Quantities	Calories
Golden Syrup	1 oz	40	100 g	142
Iced Top Christmas	,,	71	,,	250
Jamaica Ginger	,,	38	,,	134
Kensington No.2	,,	97	,,	343
Kensington Pieces	,,	100	,,	354
Kensington Slab	,,	100	,,	354

MR KIPLING

Food	Quantities	Calories	Quantities	Calories
All Butter Shorties	1 oz	136	100 g	480
Almond Slices	,,	106	,,	375
Angel Layer Cake	,,	116	,,	407
Apple Bakewell Tart	,,	104	,,	368
Apple Pies	,,	100	,,	352
Apple & Blackcurrant Pies	,,	96	,,	340
Apple Sundaes	,,	111	,,	391
Bakewell Tart	,,	115	,,	405
Bakewell Slices	,,	126	,,	443
Battenburg	,,	101	,,	357
Battenburg Treats	,,	123	,,	433
Blackcurrant Sundaes	,,	111	,,	392
Buttercream Walnut Cake	,,	125	,,	442
Cherry Bakewells	,,	116	,,	409
Cherry Fruit Cake	,,	93	,,	326
Cherry Slices	,,	114	,,	400
Cherry Walnut Slices	,,	126	,,	443
Chocolate Fudge Cake	,,	95	,,	334
Chocolate Sponge	,,	105	,,	371

Cakes, Pies, Cake Mixes, Pastries & Rolls

Food	Quantities	Calories	Quantities	Calories
Chocolate Swiss Roll	1 oz	104	100 g	368
Coconut Macaroons	"	112	"	396
Coffee Gateau	"	109	"	383
Country Slices	"	105	"	370
Dundee Cake	"	88	"	310
French Fancies	"	104	"	368
French Jam Sponge	"	98	"	346
Individual Apple Pie	"	98	"	346
Individual Apple & blackcurrant Pie	"	87	"	305
Jaffa Fingers	"	121	"	426
Jam Swiss Roll	"	86	"	302
Jam Tarts	"	105	"	370
Madeira Cake	"	109	"	383
Manor House Cake	"	95	"	334
Mince Pies	"	105	"	369
Sultana Cake	"	104	"	368
Treacle Tarts	"	100	"	351
PREWETT				
Christmas Cake, Wholemeal	1 oz	97	100 g	342
Christmas Pudding, Wholemeal	"	87	"	306
Flapjacks				
Carob & Nut	each	130	100 g	488
Date	1 oz	124	"	465
Fruit & Nut	"	125	"	469

Food	Quantities	Calories	Quantities	Calories
Oatmeal	1 oz	127	100 g	478
Mince Pie, Wholemeal	"	100	"	354
Pastry Cases	"	138	"	488

SAFEWAY
(large cakes)

Food	Quantities	Calories	Quantities	Calories
Baked Raspberry Jam Roll	1 oz	116	100 g	408
Butter Iced Fruit Bar	"	105	"	371
Cherry Cake	"	89	"	315
Cherry Genoa	"	90	"	318
Cherry Genoa, All Butter	"	95	"	335
Cherry Genoa Cut Cake	"	90	"	318
Chocolate Chip Cake	"	105	"	371
Choc Log with Buttercream	"	121	"	428
Chocolate Sponge Sandwich	"	109	"	384
Chocolate Gateau with Blackcurrant	"	105	"	369
Christmas Cake with Marzipan	"	110	"	389
Coconut Cake	"	108	"	382
Coconut Gateau & Buttercream	"	106	"	374
Dundee Cake	"	89	"	312
Dundee Cake, All Butter	"	108	"	382
Dundee Cut Cake	"	89	"	312
Giant Yule Log	"	121	"	428
Madeira Cake	"	103	"	364

Cakes, Pies, Cake Mixes, Pastries & Rolls

Food	Quantities	Calories	Quantities	Calories
Praline Gateau & Apricot	1 oz	101	100 g	356
Rich Fruit Christmas Cake	"	106	"	375
Sponge				
Blackcurrant				
w/Buttercream	"	108	"	380
Coconut w/Buttercream	"	122	"	430
Raspberry w/Buttercream	"	108	"	380
Sultana Cake	"	102	"	360
Sultana Cut Cake	"	102	"	360
(small cakes)				
Apple Dessert Pies	"	99	"	350
Apple Sundaes	"	110	"	386
Blackcurrant & Apple				
Sundaes	"	111	"	390
Bramley Apple Pies	"	96	"	338
Chocolate Mini Rolls	"	127	"	449
Deep Mince Pies	"	108	"	380
Meringue Nests	"	89	"	312
Mini Blackcurrant Pies	"	107	"	377
Sponge Fingers	"	123	"	433
Trifle Sponges	"	92	"	325
SAINSBURY				
Almond Slice	each	130		
Angel	1 oz	115	100 g	405
Bakewell Tart	"	117	"	412
Battenburg	"	103	"	362

Cakes, Pies, Cake Mixes, Pastries & Rolls

Food	Quantities	Calories	Quantities	Calories
Battenbrug, Strawberry	1 oz	100	100 g	351
Butter Walnut Sandwich	"	103	"	362
Cherry Bakewell	each	180		
Chocolate	1 oz	120	100 g	422
Chocolate Cup	each	129		
Chocolate Sandwich	1 oz	100	100 g	351
Corn Crisp	"	120	"	422
Eccles Cake	each	150		
Fondant Fancy	"	95		
Fruity Crisp	1 oz	120	100 g	422
Genoa	"	113	"	398
Iced Fruit	"	92	"	324
Jam Tart	each	140		
Madeira	1 oz	113	100 g	398
Meringue Nest	each	55		
Short Pastry Mince Pie	"	160		
Sponge Sandwich	1 oz	107	100 g	377
Strawberry Jam Sponge	11	103	"	362
Swiss Rolls				
Black Cherry				
& Buttercream	"	93	"	327
Chocolate Buttercream	"	100	"	351
Chocolate Flavoured	"	110	"	387
Jam Roll	"	80	"	282
Junior Chocolate	each	128		
Treacle Tart				
large	1 oz	104	100 g	366

Cakes, Pies, Cake Mixes, Pastries & Rolls

Food	Quantities	Calories	Quantities	Calories
small	each	155		
Trifle Sponge	each	80		
Wholemeal Carrot & Orange	1 oz	104	100 g	367
Wholemeal Harvest Fruit	,,	104	,,	365
(Rolls etc)				
Bath Buns	each	165		
Chelsea Buns	,,	195		
Chocolatines	,,	205		
Croissants	,,	200		
Crumpets	,,	75		
Currant Buns	,,	150		
Danish Pastry	,,	360		
Doughnuts	,,	215		
Fruit Scones	,,	235		
Fruited Lardy Cake	1 oz	126	100 g	445
Muffins				
Plain	each	155		
Cheese & Chive	,,	155		
Wholemeal	,,	155		
Wholemeal & Raisin	,,	140		
Pancakes				
Lemon & Raisin	,,	90		
Orange & Lemon	,,	90		
Scotch	,,	85		
Scotch, Wholemeal	,,	75		
Spiced Fruit Bun	,,	175		
Teacakes	,,	130		

Cakes, Pies, Cake Mixes, Pastries & Rolls

Food	Quantities	Calories	Quantities	Calories
Teacakes	each	130		
Wholemeal Scones	”	180		
Wholemeal Spiced Buns	”	175		
SPAR				
Apricot Fruit Pies	1 oz	110	100 g	389
Blackcurrant & Apple Pies	”	110	”	389
Bramley Apple Pies	”	110	”	389
Coconut Decorated Cake	”	123	”	435
Corn Crisp Cakes	”	134	”	472
Rice Crisp Cakes	”	135	”	475
Trifle Sponge Cakes	”	94	”	330
VIOTA *(cake mixes)*				
Carnival Cakes	1 oz	110	100 g	393
Chocolate Cup Cakes				
with water icing	”	96	”	343
with fudge topping	”	117	”	418
Chocolate Fudge Cake	”	104	”	371
Coconut Iced Cake	”	120	”	429
Coconut Macaroons	”	126	”	450
Dairy Fudge Cake	”	116	”	414
Madeira Cake	”	98	”	350
Tea Cakes	”	118	”	421
'Economix Range'				
Chocolate Sandwich Cake				
(no filling)	”	112	”	400
Crumble	”	122	”	436

Cakes, Pies, Cake Mixes, Pastries & Rolls

Food	Quantities	Calories	Quantities	Calories
Ginger Cake	1 oz	109	100 g	391
Rock Cakes	"	94	"	336
Scones	"	108	"	385
Small Cakes (no icing)	"	115	"	410
Sponge Cakes (no filling)	"	118	"	421
Yorkshire Pudding	"	91	"	325

WAITROSE
(large cakes)

Food	Quantities	Calories	Quantities	Calories
All Butter Coconut	1 oz	106	100 g	375
All Butter Madeira	"	105	"	370
Angel Sandwich	"	115	"	406
Battenberg	"	103	"	362
Black Cherry Buttercream Roll	"	102	"	360
Black Forest Gateau	"	69	"	244
Black Forest Slice	"	68	"	240
Cherry Genoa	"	106	"	372
Chocolate Buttercream Roll	"	108	"	380
Chocolate Cream Gateau	"	73	"	259
Chocolate Pavlova	"	85	"	300
Chocolate Sandwich	"	130	"	457
Chorley	"	119	"	420
Farmhouse	"	102	"	359
French Jam Sandwich	"	113	"	399
Iced Madeira Sandwich	"	120	"	423
Lemon Curd & Buttercream Roll	"	102	"	360

Cakes, Pies, Cake Mixes, Pastries & Rolls

Food	Quantities	Calories	Quantities	Calories
Lemon Soufflé	1 oz	71	100 g	250
Madeira	,,	124	,,	437
Milk Chocolate Covered Roll	,,	121	,,	428
Paradise Cake	,,	100	,,	352
Pear Helene Slice	,,	61	,,	215
Plate Apple Pie	,,	89	,,	314
Raspberry Baked Roll	,,	101	,,	356
Raspberry Cream Gateau	,,	75	,,	263
Rich Fruit	,,	100	,,	354
Sultana & Ginger Roll	,,	91	,,	320
Summer Fruit Lattice Pie	,,	96	,,	340
Treacle Baked Roll	,,	108	,,	379
Trifle Sponge	,,	88	,,	309
Tropical Fruit Lattice Pie	,,	96	,,	340
Whole Sultana	,,	98	,,	347
(small cakes)				
All Butter Eccles	,,	111	,,	390
Chocolate Topped Orange	,,	108	,,	381
Eclairs	,,	116	,,	410
Junior Rolls (jam filling)	,,	82	,,	290
Mince Pies	,,	105	,,	369
Mini Apple Pies	,,	107	,,	377
Mini Blackcurrant Pies	,,	107	,,	377
Milk Chocolate Rolls				
raspberry filling	,,	104	,,	365
vanilla filling	,,	129	,,	453
Peanut Butter Cookies	,,	85	,,	300

Cakes, Pies, Cake Mixes, Pastries & Rolls

Food	Quantities	Calories	Quantities	Calories
Puff Pastry Mince Pies	1 oz	111	100 g	391
Profiteroles	"	121	"	425
Treacle Tarts	"	105	"	370
Wholemeal Apple Pies	"	99	"	349
Wholemeal Blackcurrant Pies	"	107	"	374
Wholemeal Mince Pies	"	114	"	401

Cereals

Contrary to what we were led to believe in the past, breakfast cereals are — in the main — nutritionally healthy and not particularly fattening if weighed carefully and eaten in reasonable quantities. Clearly you must avoid those with added sugar and sweeten them only with artificial sweeteners. Also they should be served with skimmed milk, the sort with added calcium if available.

Food	Quantities	Calories	Quantities	Calories
ALLINSON				
Bran Muesli	1 oz	93	100 g	328
Bran Plus	,,	62	,,	219
Broad Bran	,,	52	,,	184
Breakfast Muesli	,,	100	,,	354
Stabilized Wheatgerm	,,	.98	,,	347
BOOTS				
'Second Nature'				
Bran Oat Crunch	1 oz	104	100 g	367

Cereals

Food	Quantities	Calories	Quantities	Calories
High Fibre Porridge	1 oz	95	100 g	335
Honey Muesli	"	118	"	417
Muesli	"	102	"	361
No Added Sugar Muesli	"	103	"	362
GRANOSE				
Bircher Muesli	1 oz	107	100 g	379
Crunchy Nut Cereal	"	139	"	493
'8' Fruit Muesli	"	115	"	408
Fruit Bran	"	85	"	302
Soya Bran	"	28	"	100
Wholegrain Fruit Muesli	"	115	"	408
HOLLAND & BARRETT				
Bran 'n' Apple Crunchy				
Cereal	1 oz	104	100 g	367
Carribean Crunchy Creal	"	111	"	390
Honey Crunchy Cereal	"	111	"	390
Muesli				
De Luxe	"	61	"	214
High Fibre	"	96	"	338
Sugar Free	"	108	"	380
Nutty Crunchy Cereal	"	102	"	361
HOLLY MILLS				
Bran Breakfast	1 oz	124	100 g	441
Bran B'Fast with				
Apple & Banana	"	124	"	438

Food	Quantities	Calories	Quantities	Calories
Crunchy Cereal	1 oz	117	100 g	415
Fruit & Nut Porridge	”	98	”	347
Honey Toasted Wheatflakes	”	92	”	326
Muesli				
Base	”	100	”	351
de Luxe	”	102	”	362
Paradise	”	94	”	332
Sugar Free	”	98	”	346
KALIBU				
De-Luxe Muesli	1 oz	110	100 g	390
Fruit & Nut Muesli				
KELLOGG				
All-Bran	1 oz	71	100 g	249
Bran Buds	”	77	”	271
Bran Flakes	”	86	”	302
Coco Pops	”	102	”	358
Corn Flakes	”	99	”	350
Crunchy Nut Corn Flakes	”	107	”	378
Frosties	”	101	”	355
Fruit ’n’ Fibre	”	96	”	338
Honey Smacks	”	98	”	346
Nutri-Grain				
Brown Rice & Rye	”	95	”	336
Rye & Oats	”	106	”	372
Whole Wheat with Raisins	”	92	”	325

Cereals

Food	Quantities	Calories	Quantities	Calories
Rice Krispies	1 oz	100	100 g	351
Ricicles	"	100	"	351
Special K	"	101	"	355
Start	"	96	"	340
Sultana Bran	"	85	"	298
Summer Orchard	"	91	"	320
JORDAN				
Muesli				
Country	1 oz	97	100 g	345
Special Recipe				
Natural Country Bran	"	54	"	190
Natural Wheatgerm	"	95	"	337
'Original Crunchy Cereal'				
Bran & Apple	"	104	"	369
Honey, Almonds & Raisins	"	112	"	396
Natural	"	114	"	405
Original Recipe	"	117	"	416
LYONS				
Coco Brek	1 oz	110	100 g	388
Golden Brek	"	111	"	391
Ready Brek Original	"	111	"	391
MARKS & SPENCER				
Banana Bran Flakes	1 oz	98	100 g	345
Bran Muesli – unsweetened	"	96	"	337

Food	Quantities	Calories	Quantities	Calories
Breakfast Special	1 oz	98	100 g	347
Cornflakes & Wheatflakes	”	100	”	354
Honey Crisp Rice	”	100	”	352
Muesli				
Traditional	”	103	”	362
Unsweetened	”	96	”	340
PREWETT				
Jumbo Oats	1 oz	105	100 g	370
Muesli				
Base	”	96	”	338
Bran	”	93	”	328
De Luxe	”	107	”	378
Fruit & Nut	”	96	”	339
Honey	”	93	”	329
Tropical	”	100	”	354
QUAKER				
'Harvest Crunch'				
Bran & Apple	1 oz	121	100 g	425
Sultanas, Raisin	”	127	”	446
Oat Krunchies	”	109	”	383
Puffed Wheat	”	92	”	325
Quaker Oats	”	107	”	377
Warm Start	”	105	”	370
SAFEWAY				
Cornflakes	1 oz	100	100 g	352

Cereals

Food	Quantities	Calories	Quantities	Calories
Crunchy Cereal	1 oz	118	100 g	415
Fibre Bran	"	70	"	248
Fruit & Nut Muesli, 35%	"	93	"	326
Hot Oat Cereal	"	109	"	384
Quick Cooking Oats	"	107	"	377
Rice Crunchies	"	100	"	352
Swiss Style Cereal	"	94	"	330
Whole Wheat				
Breakfast Biscuits	"	98	"	344
Whole Wheat Flakes	"	92	"	325
SAINSBURY				
Bran Flakes	1 oz	90	100 g	318
Cocosnaps	"	100	"	351
Cornflakes	"	90	"	318
Crunchy Oat Cereal	"	119	"	418
Crunchy Oat Cereal w/Bran	"	114	"	368
Honey Nut Cornflakes	"	100	"	351
Instant Hot Oat Cereal	"	114	"	368
Instant Hot Oat Cereal				
w/Bran	"	114	"	368
Mini Wheats	"	95	"	334
Oat & Bran Flakes	"	85	"	301
Puffed Wheat	"	90	"	318
Rice Pops	"	100	"	351
Snowflakes	"	100	"	351
Sultana Bran	"	85	"	301

Cereals

Food	Quantities	Calories	Quantities	Calories
Swiss Style Muesli	1 oz	91	100 g	321
Toasted Bran	"	85	"	301
Wheat Flakes	"	.95	"	334
Wholewheat Bisk	2 biscuits	210		
Wholewheat Mini Flakes	1 oz	.85	100 g	301

SPAR

Food	Quantities	Calories	Quantities	Calories
Cornflakes	1 oz	99	100 g	350
Swiss Style Muesli	"	91	"	320

WAITROSE

Food	Quantities	Calories	Quantities	Calories
Bran Flakes	1 oz	96	100 g	340
Bran Muesli	"	103	"	363
Cornflakes	"	98	"	345
Crunchy Cornflakes w/Honey & Nuts	"	116	"	410
Fruit & Nut Muesli	"	83	"	293
Oat Crunchy – all flavours	"	111	"	390
Porridge Oats	"	101	"	355
Rice Crunchies	"	99	"	350
Wheat Bran	"	70	"	248
Wheat Flakes	"	.95	"	335

Crisps & Savoury Snacks

There has been a particularly great increase in the number of products available in this category since the last edition of this book was compiled. There is now particular emphasis on absence of artificial flavourings and colour, on use of wholewheat flour and on lower fat content. All this makes it possible for the dieter to enjoy the occasional between-meal snack without irreparably damaging his or her health but does not make any difference to the calorie-count! The number of different flavours on the market now is quite remarkable.

Food	Quantities	Calories	Quantities	Calories
CADBURY				
Criss Cross	1 oz	129	100 g	454
Stackers	"	128	"	450

Food	Quantities	Calories	Quantities	Calories
GOLDEN WONDER				
Stix				
'Bigger Bite'				
Cheese & Onion	1 pkt (25g)	115		
Prawn Cocktail	"	120		
Salt & Vinegar	"	117		
Tortilla Chips	1 oz	146	100 g	513
Wotsits				
Cheesy	1 pkt	128		
Barbequed Beef	"	111		
Cheese/Bacon	"	114		
Tomato	"	111		
Crisps				
Barbecued Beef	1 pkt (28g)	139		
Cheese & Onion	"	141		
Crispy Bacon	"	140		
Oxo	"	123		
Prawn Cocktail	"	139		
Ready salted	"	142		
Roast Chicken	"	139		
Salt & Vinegar	"	139		
Savoury Sausage	"	140		
Spring Onion	"	140		
Worcestershire Sauce	"	124		
Crackles	1 pkt (17g)	87		
Oddums				
Barbequed Beef	1 pkt (24g)	112		

Crisps & Savoury Snacks

Food	Quantities	Calories	Quantities	Calories
Cheeseburger	1 pkt (24g)	116		
Salt & Vinegar	"	115		
Preludes				
Cheese	1 oz	151	100 g	533
Herb	"	145	"	509
Pizza	"	158	"	558
Sesame	"	146	"	514
Wafer Thin	"	143	"	504
Ringos				
Cheese & Onion	1 pkt (21g)	97		
Mild Curry	"	96		
Salt & Vinegar	"	96		
Steak & Onion	"	95		
Stix				
Cheese & Onion	1 pkt (26g)	115		
Prawn Cocktail	"	114		
Ready Salted	"	117		
Salt & Vinegar	"	114		
HOLLAND & BARRETT				
Millet Flakes	1 oz	89	100 g	313
Pumpkin Seeds	"	164	"	579
Sesame Seeds	"	165	"	582
Sunflower Seeds	"	165	"	582
HOLLY MILLS				
'Mumbo Jumbos'				
Cheese & Leek	1 pkt (20g)	90	100 g	450

Food	Quantities	Calories	Quantities	Calories
Chilli	1 pkt (20g)	90	100 g	450
Plain	,,	90	,,	450

MARKS & SPENCER

Food	Quantities	Calories	Quantities	Calories
Barbecue Spare Rib Crisps	1 oz	148	100 g	520
Burger Bites	,,	156	,,	550
Cocktail Crisps	,,	156	,,	550
Corn Chips – Californian	,,	162	,,	570
Crinkles	,,	150	,,	530
Crisps				
Barbecue Beef & Onion	,,	151	,,	531
Beef, lower fat	,,	135	,,	476
Chargrill Beef	,,	151	,,	532
Cheese & Onion	,,	148	,,	520
Cheese/Onion, lower fat	,,	136	,,	480
Ready Salted	,,	156	,,	550
Ready Salted, low fat	,,	138	,,	485
Salt & Vinegar	,,	150	,,	530
Spring Onion	,,	155	,,	546
Deltas	,,	137	,,	484
Pizza Bits – Italian Style	,,	134	,,	473
Potato Rings	,,	146	,,	516
Potato Waffles	,,	131	,,	463
Prawn Cocktail Snacks	,,	148	,,	520
Prawn Crackers	,,	123	,,	435
Ready Salted Potato Sticks	,,	144	,,	508
Ready Salted Potato Thins	,,	134	,,	472

Crisps & Savoury Snacks

Food	Quantities	Calories	Quantities	Calories
Salt & Vinegar Chiplets	1 oz	137	100 g	481
Scamps	"	140	"	493
Tortilla Chips	"	141	"	498
PREWETT'S				
Savoury Hungarian	1 pkt	163	100 g	326
Spicy Mexican	"	160	"	319
Tasty Italian	"	163	"	326
PROTOVEG				
Natural	1 oz	82	100 g	288
Flavoured	"	79	"	280
Smoky Snaps	"	126	"	443
SAFEWAY				
Bacon Streaks	1 oz	133	100 g	470
Carnival Mix	"	96	"	337
Crinkle Cut Crisps	"	152	"	534
Crisps – all flavours	"	142	"	500
Crispy Squares	"	134	"	472
Crispy Squares, Salt & Vinegar	"	131	"	460
Crunchy Sticks	"	137	"	483
Crunchy Sticks, Salt & Vinegar	"	137	"	483
Onion Rings	"	142	"	500
Potato Sticks	"	143	"	505

Food	Quantities	Calories	Quantities	Calories
Potato Twirls	1 oz	123	100 g	434
Savoury Puffs	,,	171	,,	602
Savoury Twigs	,,	111	,,	391
Trail Mix	,,	141	,,	495
Tropical Mix	,,	127	,,	446
Wheat Crunchies	,,	137	,,	482

SAINSBURY

Cheese & Ham Nibbles	1 bag	130		
Cheese & Onion Potato Crisps	,,	140		
Cheese Flavoured Potato Snacks	,,	133		
Cheese Flavoured Puffs	,,	150		
Cheese Savouries	each	4		
Crunchy Sticks	1 bag	120		
Ocean Crunchies	1 bag	125		
Onion Rings	,,	125		
Potato Chips	,,	125		
Potato Crisps	,,	135		
Potato Rings	,,	130		
Potato Squares	,,	115		
Prawn Cocktail Snacks	,,	125		
Salt & Vinegar Potato Sticks	,,	120		
Twiglets	each	3		

SOONER

Caribbean Cocktail	1 oz	143	100 g	503

Crisps & Savoury Snacks

Food	Quantities	Calories	Quantities	Calories
Cashews	1 oz	159	100 g	560
Crisps	ʺ	151	ʺ	533
Crunchy Coated Peanuts	ʺ	139	ʺ	490
Dry Roast Peanuts	ʺ	171	ʺ	602
Harvest Rings	ʺ	129	ʺ	453
Mixed Nuts & Raisins	ʺ	139	ʺ	488
Nik-Naks	ʺ	141	ʺ	497
Plain Peanuts & Raisins	ʺ	135	ʺ	476
Salted Peanuts	ʺ	162	ʺ	572
SPAR				
Alphas	1 oz	137	100 g	484
Beasties Pickled Onion	ʺ	131	ʺ	460
Burger Bites	ʺ	156	ʺ	549
Cheesey Curls	ʺ	145	ʺ	511
Cheesy Puffs	ʺ	169	ʺ	594
Cheesies	ʺ	164	ʺ	574
Crisps				
Assorted 6-pack	ʺ	148	ʺ	520
Beef	ʺ	153	ʺ	534
Cheese & Onion	ʺ	151	ʺ	532
Ready Salted	ʺ	156	ʺ	550
Salt & Vinegar	ʺ	149	ʺ	526
Crispy Squares	ʺ	135	ʺ	472
Crunchy Fries	ʺ	125	ʺ	440
Crunchy Sticks	ʺ	137	ʺ	483
Genies Barbeque Flavour	ʺ	135	ʺ	474

Food	Quantities	Calories	Quantities	Calories
Onion Rings	1 oz	142	100 g	500
Potato Rings	,,	146	,,	516
Potato Sticks Barbeque	,,	141	,,	493
Potato Sticks, ready salted	,,	144	,,	508
Prawn Cocktail Snacks	,,	148	,,	520
WAITROSE				
Bacon Snacks	1 oz	139	100 g	490
Caribbean Mix	,,	132	,,	465
Cheese Flavoured Savoury Puffs	,,	149	,,	526
Cheese Twists	,,	132	,,	465
Cheese Savouries	,,	147	,,	517
Crispy Thins	,,	137	,,	484
Exotic Fruit & Nuts	,,	126	,,	445
Fruit, Nuts & Seeds	,,	133	,,	470
Onion Rings	,,	137	,,	483
Party Twigs	,,	113	,,	399
Potato Crisps – all Flavours	,,	148	,,	520
Potato Rings	,,	146	,,	516
Potato Sticks	,,	144	,,	508
Prawn Cocktail Snacks	,,	148	,,	520
Salt & Vinegar Potato Twirls	,,	120	,,	423
Salt & Vinegar Savoury Sticks	,,	137	,,	483
Salted Pistachio Nuts	,,	179	,,	630
Wheat Crunchies	,,	137	,,	482

Crisps & Savoury Snacks

Food	Quantities	Calories	Quantities	Calories
WHEATEATS				
Cheese	1 pkt	111	100 g	444
Chilli	"	102	"	410
Natural	"	102	"	407
Onion	"	107	"	428
Peanut Butter	"	123	"	490
Pizza	"	111	"	428

Dairy Products, Fats, Oils & Non Dairy Substitutes

This section has been rearranged in this new edition as there are so many more products now in this category, including such exotic items as 'Brandy Cream' and 'Vegetarian Cheese'! Cheeses have been listed first, and not under brand-name as the calorie content does not vary. This excludes processed cheeses and flavoured cottage cheese. Some non-dairy products which have been produced as substitutes for dairy ones are listed, as in the last edition. This list is not, unfortunately, complete as it was difficult to obtain the information. It is believed that this is printed on the packets in many cases.

Food	Quantities	Calories	Quantities	Calories
CHEESE, HARD *(average, all brands)*				
Caerphilly	1 oz	105	100 g	370
Cheddar	,,	120	,,	420

Dairy Products, Fats, Oils & Non Dairy Substitutes

Food	Quantities	Calories	Quantities	Calories
Cheshire	1 oz	110	100 g	388
Danish Blue	,,	114	,,	400
Derby	,,	110	,,	388
Double Gloucester	,,	110	,,	388
Edam	,,	90	,,	320
Emmenthal	,,	105	,,	370
Gorgonzola	,,	112	,,	395
Gouda	,,	96	,,	340
Gruyere	,,	120	,,	420
Jarlsberg	,,	100	,,	350
Lancashire	,,	100	,,	350
Leicester	,,	110	,,	390
Parmesan	,,	120	,,	416
Port Salut	,,	90	,,	315
Smoked	,,	110	,,	390
St. Paulin	,,	85	,,	300
Stilton	,,	135	,,	480
Wensleydale	,,	110	,,	390
Cheese, soft				
Boursin	,,	115	,,	404
Blue Brie	,,	123	,,	435
Bressot	,,	74	,,	262
Camembert	,,	.75	,,	265
Curd	,,	35	,,	123
Edelweiss	,,	111	,,	393
Quark	,,	25	,,	88

Dairy Products, Fats, Oils & Non Dairy Substitutes

Food	Quantities	Calories	Quantities	Calories
BIRD'S EYE *(frozen)*				
Whipped Dairy Cream	1 fl oz	60	100 ml	211
BUITONI				
Parmesan Cheese (grated)	1 oz	140	100 g	494
CADBURY				
Coffee Compliment	1 portion	10	100 g	540
Marvel	"	10	"	355
CARNATION				
Coffee Mate	1 tsp	10	100 g	535
Evaporated Milk	1 oz	45	"	160
CHAMBOURCY				
Cottage Cheese				
natural	1 oz	31	100 g	109
with Chives	"	30	"	108
with Pineapple	"	29	"	104
Cream				
double	1 fl. oz	127	100 ml	449
single	"	54	"	189
whipping	"	94	"	332
Yoghurt				
'Bonjour'				
Exotic Fruits	1 oz	21	100 g	74
Lemon	"	21	"	74

Dairy Products, Fats, Oils & Non Dairy Substitutes

Food	Quantities	Calories	Quantities	Calories
Strawberry	1 oz	14	100 g	51
Vanilla	"	22	"	78
'Nouvelle'				
Black Cherry	1 oz	22	100 g	78
Kiwi & Gooseberry	"	22	"	78
Peach & Redcurrant	"	22	"	78
Raspberry	"	21	"	73
Rhubarb	"	23	"	80
'Robot'				
Black Cherry	"	21	"	73
Banana	"	22	"	78
Raspberry	"	21	"	73
Strawberry	"	22	"	78
'Whole Milk'				
Apricot	"	29	"	102
Fruits of the Forest	"	28	"	100
Strawberry	"	27	"	97
DOVE'S FARM				
Soft Fresh Goat's Cheese all varieties	75 g pot	169	100 g	225
EDENVALE				
Cottage Cheese				
Apricot & Apple	1 oz	26	100 g	92
Celery & Blue Cheese	"	26	"	92
Cheddar & Onion	"	34	"	121

Dairy Products, Fats, Oils & Non Dairy Substitutes

Food	Quantities	Calories	Quantities	Calories
Crunchy	1 oz	32	100 g	112
Natural	"	27	"	97
Onion & Chive	"	27	"	97
Pineapple	"	28	"	98
Salmon & Cucumber	"	31	"	110
Seafood	"	26	"	92
'Diet' average all flavours	"	23	"	83
Cream				
Clotted	1 fl. oz	145	100 ml	510
Double & U.H.T.	"	128	"	450
Half Cream, U.H.T.	"	39	"	136
Single & U.H.T.	"	.54	"	190
Soured	"	54	"	190
Spooning	"	103	"	363
Whipping & U.H.T.	"	103	"	363
Soft Cheese 'Somerset'				
high fat	1 oz	91	100 g	321
low fat	"	.38	"	135
medium fat Cucumber	"	56	"	196
medium fat Onion & Gherkin	"	57	"	201
medium fat Pineapple	"	58	"	206
Yoghurt				
Apple	"	29	"	102
Banana	"	28	"	99
Blackberry	"	27	"	95
Chocolate	"	31	"	108

Dairy Products, Fats, Oils & Non Dairy Substitutes

Food	Quantities	Calories	Quantities	Calories
French Style	1 oz	25	100 g	87
Fudge	,,	26	,,	92
Natural	,,	20	,,	70
Raspberry	,,	28	,,	99
Sherbert Lemon	,,	26	,,	92
Strawberry	,,	28	,,	100
ELMLEA				
Longlife Cream				
single	1 tbs	28	100 ml	195
whipping	,,	45	,,	330
FUSSELLS *(tinned)*				
Condensed Milk	1 oz	76	100 g	267
Golden Butterfly Cream	,,	66	,,	233
GRANOSE (non-dairy)				
Margarine				
low salt	1 oz	212	100 g	750
plain	,,	212	,,	750
sunflower	,,	203	,,	720
Soya Desserts				
Chocolate	,,	22	,,	77
Strawberry	,,	20	,,	72
Vanilla	,,	20	,,	72
Soya Milk				
Carob	,,	17	,,	59

Dairy Products, Fats, Oils & Non Dairy Substitutes

Food	Quantities	Calories	Quantities	Calories
Coconut	1 oz	20	100 g	70
Plain	"	14	"	50
Strawberry	"	18	"	64
Soyagen, powdered Soya Milk	"	140	"	496
KRAFT				
Butter				
Golden Churn	1 oz	193	100 g	680
Cheese				
Cheddar Slices	"	93	"	326
Cheddar Spread	"	79	"	277
Cheddar & Blue Spread	"	77	"	273
Cheshire Slices	"	95	"	335
Cracker Barrel	"	115	"	406
Margarine				
Plain	"	207	"	730
Superfine Soft tub	"	207	"	730
Vitalite Sunflower	"	207	"	730
Lard & Cooking Fat (average)	1 oz	262	25 g	230
LCD				
Yoghurt 'Fruit of the Forest'				
Blackberry	1 oz	82	100 g	288
Blackcurrant	"	81	"	287
Cherry	"	84	"	295
Strawberry	"	81	"	287

Dairy Products, Fats, Oils & Non Dairy Substitutes

Food	Quantities	Calories	Quantities	Calories
LOSELEY				
Cottage Cheese	1 oz	38	100 g	133
Cream				
double	1 fl. oz	125	100 ml	440
single	,,	63	,,	221
soured	,,	54	,,	192
whipping	,,	103	,,	364
Lebnie	,,	33	,,	118
Yoghurt				
Apricot	1 oz	18	100 g	65
Banana	,,	24	,,	85
Black Cherry	,,	21	,,	76
Blackcurrant	,,	22	,,	85
Greek Style	,,	41	,,	143
Hazelnut	,,	28	,,	100
Natural	,,	11	,,	40
Raspberry	,,	23	,,	81
Strawberry	,,	21	,,	76
MARKS & SPENCER				
Brandy Sauce	1 oz	35	100 g	123
Butter				
Brandy	,,	152	,,	537
Cornish	,,	210	,,	740
English Churn	,,	194	,,	682
Cream				
Brandy, thick double	1 fl. oz	123	100 ml	435

Dairy Products, Fats, Oils & Non Dairy Substitutes

Food	Quantities	Calories	Quantities	Calories
Brandy, whippped	1 fl. oz	122	100 ml	430
Cornish Clotted	"	162	"	570
double	"	128	"	450
fresh thick 30%	"	84	"	295
fresh thick double	"	128	"	450
half	"	40	"	140
single	"	60	"	212
single U.H.T.	"	54	"	190
thick Rum double	"	125	"	439
whiskey double, thick	"	125	"	440
whipping	"	108	"	380
Cheese, Processed				
dairy	1 oz	85	100 g	300
process cheddar slices	"	96	"	340
spread with Walnuts	"	88	"	310
Cheese, soft				
Cottage				
Apple, Celery, Nut	"	45	"	157
Chicken & Asparagus	"	42	"	147
Chicken, Tuna, Sweetcorn,				
Pepper	"	43	"	151
Natural Lite	"	20	"	70
Creamy & Prawns	"	50	"	175
Creamy, natural	"	38	"	133
Prawn Snack	"	46	"	163
w/Pineapple	"	34	"	120
w/Prawns	"	47	"	166

Dairy Products, Fats, Oils & Non Dairy Substitutes

Food	Quantities	Calories	Quantities	Calories
Beef, Horseradish	1 oz	42	100 g	147
Salmon Cucumber	″	36	″	126
Full Fat Soft	″	70	″	248
Goat	″	89	″	315
Custard Sauce	″	34	″	120
Spreads				
Golden	″	202	″	710
Lite Low Fat	″	105	″	370
Sunflower Margarine	″	207	″	730
Yoghurt				
Apricot & Guava	″	31	″	109
Apricot & Passion Fruit	″	28	″	100
Black Cherry	″	31	″	110
Cherry & Apricot	″	30	″	105
French Style & 4 pack	″	24	″	85
Lemon	″	29	″	103
Strawberry	″	29	″	103
Greengage & Gooseberry	″	24	″	85
Natural	″	17	″	59
Nectarines & Orange	″	28	″	98
Peach Melba	″	27	″	94
Pineapple & Grapefruit	″	30	″	106
Raspberry & Passion Fruit	″	33	″	115
Raspberry Ripple	″	36	″	126
Rhubarb	″	26	″	92
Strawberry & Wild Herb	″	33	″	117
Strawberry	″	27	″	95

Dairy Products, Fats, Oils & Non Dairy Substitutes

Food	Quantities	Calories	Quantities	Calories
Sunfruit	1 oz	29	100 g	104
Thick & Creamy				
Fruits of Forest	,,	32	,,	113
Toffee	,,	32	,,	112
Whole Milk Natural				
French	,,	19	,,	68
'Lite' – all flavours	,,	11	,,	39
MATTESON				
Cottage Cheese				
plain	1 oz	16	100 g	56
with Chives	,,	16	,,	56
with Pineapple	,,	19	,,	67
NESTLES (tinned)				
Cream	1 oz	66	100 g	233
Milk				
condensed	,,	92	,,	325
evaporated	,,	45	,,	160
Oil				
Corn (average)	1 fl. oz	208	25 ml	200
Olive (average)	,,	252	,,	220
Sunflower &				
Safflower	,,	208	,,	200
Soya	,,	208	,,	200
Vegetable (average)	,,	255	,,	225

Dairy Products, Fats, Oils & Non Dairy Substitutes

Food	Quantities	Calories	Quantities	Calories
PHILADELPHIA				
Cream Cheese				
light	1 oz	56	100 g	198
plain	"	91	"	322
with chives	"	91	"	322
with garlic & herbs	"	91	"	322
PREWETT				
Soya Milk	1 fl. oz	17	100 ml	61
Vegetarian Cheese				
Bleasdale	1 oz	118	100 g	417
Cheddar	"	118	"	417
Cheshire	"	106	"	374
Double Gloucester	"	108	"	382
Fat-Reduced	"	72	"	253
Lancashire	"	104	"	366
Red Leicester	"	108	"	382
Wensleydale	"	106	"	374
SAFEWAY				
Butter				
Cornish Tub	1 oz	208	100 g	731
Devon Roll	"	208	"	731
English w/Garlic	"	200	"	704
Scan Style	"	213	"	749
Welsh w/Herbs & Garlic	"	197	"	695
Cheese				
Cheddar slices	"	85	"	300

Dairy Products, Fats, Oils & Non Dairy Substitutes

Food	Quantities	Calories	Quantities	Calories
Cottage				
Cheddar & Onion	1 oz	36	100 g	127
Chives	"	29	"	104
Date & Walnut	"	38	"	119
Onion & Pepper	"	26	"	92
Pineapple	"	28	"	98
Processed Slices	"	85	"	300
Spread Portions	"	81	"	285
Cream				
Brandy	1 fl. oz	126	100 ml	443
double	"	131	"	462
extra thick	"	127	"	447
half	"	39	"	137
Rum	"	127	"	446
single	"	54	"	190
soured	"	54	"	190
whipping	"	110	"	387
SAINSBURY				
Cheese				
Cottage				
Chives	1 oz	26	100 g	92
Cucumber, Celery & Onion	"	27	"	84
Cucumber & Cheddar	"	35	"	111
Pineapple	"	28	"	88
Salmon & Cucumber	"	37	"	115
Fromage Frais				
1% fat	"	13	"	45

Dairy Products, Fats, Oils & Non Dairy Substitutes

Food	Quantities	Calories	Quantities	Calories
8% fat	1 oz	31	100 g	110
Apricot	"	38	"	135
with Fruit	60 g pot	85	"	140
Milk 'Low Fat Flavoured'				
Banana	1 fl. oz	14	100 ml	50
Chocolate	"	17	"	60
Strawberry	"	14	"	50
Skim Milk Powder	1 tbs	5		
Yoghurt				
'Dairy Farm	1 pot	120		
'Diet'				
Blackcherry	1 pot	55		
Fruits of the Forest	"	55		
Nectarine & Apricot	"	60		
Peach Melba	"	50		
Rhubarb	"	50		
Strawberry	"	50		
French Recipe	"	100		
'Low Fat'				
Black Cherry	"	135		
Fruits of the Forest	"	145		
Hazelnut	"	150		
Lychee & Mango	"	120		
Nectarine & Apricot	"	145		
Peach Melba	"	145		
Plum	"	135		
Raspberry & Redcurrant	"	140		

Dairy Products, Fats, Oils & Non Dairy Substitutes

Food	Quantities	Calories	Quantities	Calories
Rhubarb	1 pot	120		
Strawberry	,,	130		
'Mr Men'				
Apple	,,	110		
Banana	,,	120		
Blackcherry	,,	115		
Chocolate	,,	125		
Fruits of the Forest	125 g	55		
Fudge	1 pot	125		
Peach Melba	,,	120		
Raspberry	,,	120		
Rhubarb	125 g	55		
Strawberry	1 pot	120		
'Swiss Dairy Style'				
Blackcherry & Chocolate	,,	165		
Mountain Berries	,,	155		
Strawberries	,,	140		
'Thick & Creamy'				
Apricot & Mango	,,	180		
Raspberry & Blackberry	,,	180		
Strawberry	,,	165		
ST IVEL				
Cheese				
Cheddar with Celery	1 oz	110	100 g	388
Cheddar with Herbs & Garlic	,,	116	,,	410
Cheddar with Walnuts	,,	119	,,	420

Dairy Products, Fats, Oils & Non Dairy Substitutes

Food	Quantities	Calories	Quantities	Calories
Double Gloucester with				
Chives & Onions	1 oz	114	100 g	400
Family Favourites (average)	"	79	"	280
Gold Spinner	"	79	"	280
Pizza Style	"	115	"	405
Smokey Cheddar with Paprika				
and Onion	"	116	"	410
Vegetarian	"	116	"	410
Fromage Frais				
Apricot	"	17	"	59
Strawberry	"	19	"	66
Yoghurt				
Natural Traditional – set	"	17	"	59
'Prize Italiano'				
Average all flavours	"	38	"	135
'Rainbow'				
Average all flavours	"	20	"	70
'Real'				
Average all flavours	"	23	"	82
'Shape'				
natural	"	14	"	50
average all other flavours	"	12	"	41
SKI				
Yoghurt				
Forest Fruits	1 oz	24	100 g	85
Hazelnut	"	25	"	88

Dairy Products, Fats, Oils & Non Dairy Substitutes

Food	Quantities	Calories	Quantities	Calories
Average, all other flavours	1 oz	23	100 g	82
'Diet Ski'				
Mandarin	"	16	"	56
Rhubarb	"	15	"	52
Average, all other flavours	"	16	"	55
'Gold Ski'				
Apricot & Guava	"	32	"	114
Boysenberry & Passionfruit	"	33	"	118
Forest Fruits	"	33	"	118
Strawberry	"	33	"	116
SOJAL (non-dairy)				
Dairy Free Frozen Dessert	1 serving	98	100 g	179
Soja Milk	"	108	"	43
Yoga	"	75	"	60
SPAR				
Butter	1 oz	21	"	76
Cheese				
Slices	"	21	"	76
Spread	"	21	"	76
Spread in Tubs	"	21	"	76
Cottage	"	25	"	87
'Milk Drinks'				
Banana	"	25	"	49
Chocolate	"	17	"	60
Strawberry	"	14	"	50

Dairy Products, Fats, Oils & Non Dairy Substitutes

Food	Quantities	Calories	Quantities	Calories
'Yoghurt'	1 oz	15	100 g	52
Fruits of the Forest	"	15	"	52
Grapefruit	"	25	"	87
Mandarin	"	25	"	87
Natural, unsweetened	"	15	"	52
Average, all others	"	21	"	76
SUN-PAT				
Cheddar Spread	1 oz	81	100 g	285
Dairy Spread	"	76	"	268
SWISS KNIGHT				
Cheese	1 oz	91	100 g	321
WAITROSE				
Brandy Butter	1 oz	150	100 g	530
Cream				
Brandy	1 fl. oz	126	100 ml	443
Double	"	128	"	450
Extra Thick Double	"	128	"	450
Half	"	37	"	130
Soured	"	50	"	178
Whipping	"	108	"	380
Cheese				
Cheddar Spread	"	74	"	260
Cheddar Spread with Ham,				
Prawns	"	74	"	260

Dairy Products, Fats, Oils & Non Dairy Substitutes

Food	Quantities	Calories	Quantities	Calories
Cottage				
Chedder & Onion	1 gl. oz	32	100 ml	113
Chicken & Mushroom	,,	28	,,	100
Onion & Chives	,,	24	,,	85
Pineapple & Ham	,,	27	,,	96
Prawns	,,	32	,,	112
Processed	,,	74	,,	260
Milk				
Evaporated	,,	45	,,	159
Soya	,,	12	,,	42
Spray Dried Skimmed (dry)	1 oz	101	100 g	355
Yoghurt				
'Creamy'				
Blackcurrant &				
Rose Hip	,,	41	,,	146
Fruits of the Forest	,,	41	,,	146
Raspberry & Melon	,,	38	,,	134
Strawberry	,,	40	,,	141
'Light Set French'	,,	23	,,	83
'Low Fat'				
Black Cherry	,,	27	,,	95
Champagne & Rhubarb	,,	27	,,	95
Chocolate	,,	28	,,	98
Hazelnut	,,	28	,,	98
Mandarin	,,	26	,,	93
Natural	,,	17	,,	59
Peach Melba	,,	29	,,	103

Dairy Products, Fats, Oils & Non Dairy Substitutes

Food	Quantities	Calories	Quantities	Calories
Pineapple & Coconut	1 oz	25	100 g	87
Strawberry	"	27	"	95
Average, all other flavours	"	25	"	90
WAISTLINE				
Yoghurt				
Black Cherry	1 oz	15	100 g	52
Natural	"	13	"	45
Prune	"	15	"	54
Strawberry	"	14	"	51
YOUNG'S (*frozen*)				
Cream				
Clotted	1 fl. oz	148	100 g	520
Dairy Whipping	"	94	"	330
Double	"	128	"	450
Single	"	51	"	180
Whipped	"	98	"	345

Desserts

There is a long, and extremely diverse, list of ready-to-eat desserts, as can be seen from a quick glance at this section. Clearly some are considerably lower in calories than others and these should be chosen where possible. There is no clear dividing line between 'desserts' and 'gateaux' so some appear here and others under 'cakes'. On the whole it is only the frozen ones which are listed in this section, but if you are unable to find a particular product here check in the 'cakes' section.

Food	Quantities	Calories	Quantities	Calories
AMBROSIA *(tinned)*				
Creamed Macaroni	1 oz	27	100 g	92
Creamed Rice	"	26	"	91
Creamed Sago	"	23	"	83
Creamed Semolina	"	23	"	83
Creamed Tapioca	"	23	"	83

Desserts

Food	Quantities	Calories	Quantities	Calories
Devon Custard	1 oz	28	100 g	100
Light Rice Pudding	,,	21	,,	76
Traditional Rice Pudding	,,	29	,,	102
Topsy Turvy	,,	29	,,	101
BEJAM *(frozen)*				
Black Forest Gateau	1/8 cake	235		
Chocolate Dairy				
Cream Sponge	1/6 cake	104		
Coffee/Mandarin Gateau	1/8 cake	213		
Dairy Cream Eclairs	each	103		
Dairy Cream Sponge	1/6 cake	105		
Mousse, average all				
flavours	1 tub	77		
Party Black Forest Gateau	1/14 cake	193		
Party Strawberry Gateau	,,	204		
Strawberry Gateau	1/8 cake	169		
Tropical Fruit Pavlova	1/8 cake	183		
BIRD'S EYE *(frozen)*				
Arctic Circles				
chocolate	one	165		
vanilla	,,	155		
Arctic Cup	1 tub	185		
Arctic Gateau				
Choc 'n' Cherry	1/5 cake	100		
Strawberry	,,	105		
Arctic Log	1/6 cake	100		

Food	Quantities	Calories	Quantities	Calories
Arctic Roll	1/6 small roll	75		
Black Forest Cake	1/6 cake	150		
Black Forest Dessert	1 tub	155		
Black Forest Gateau	1/6 cake	250		
Black Forest Sponge	"	120		
Cheesecake – Fruit	"	130		
Chocolate Lovely	1 tub	235		
Dairy Cream Choux Buns	one	130		
Dairy Cream & Choc. Sponge	1/6 cake	110		
Dairy Cream Doughnuts	one	170		
Dairy Cream Eclairs	"	145		
Dairy Cream Sponge	1/6 cake	130		
Melba, peach	1 tub	130		
Mousse, all flavours	"	110		
Strawberry Cream Cake	1/6 cake	145		
Strawberry Gateau	"	280		
Supermousse				
Choc'n' nut	1 tub	150		
Mint Choc. Chip	"	140		
Toffee Caramello	"	120		
all others	"	120		
Superwhip	1 level dstsp	12	1 tub	855
Trifle	1 tub	120		
BROWN & POLSON (dry)				
Blancmange				
Banana	pint sachet	124	100 g	327

Desserts

Food	Quantities	Calories	Quantities	Calories
Chocolate	pint sachet	136	100 g	335
Peach	"	125	"	330
Raspberry	"	125	"	330
Strawberry	"	125	"	330
Vanilla	"	118	"	328
Cornflour, Patent	1 oz	94	"	330
Custard Mix, instant	"	115	"	404
CHAMBOURCY				
'Chambor'				
Raspberry and Blackberry	1 oz	39	100 g	139
Tropical Fruits	"	37	"	131
'Chamby'	"	32	"	114
'Cheesecakes' – individual				
Blackcherry	"	64	"	224
Blackcurrant	"	73	"	257
Strawberry	"	77	"	271
'Creme Desserts'				
Chocolate & Vanilla	"	39	"	137
'Creme Vienna'				
Chocolate	"	37	"	132
Strawberry	"	34	"	121
'Flanby'	"	28	"	100
'Fruit Sundae'				
Cocktail	"	31	"	111
Raspberry	"	34	"	119
Tropical Fruits	"	30	"	106

Food	Quantities	Calories	Quantities	Calories
'Les Grands Desserts'				
Chocolate & Vanilla	1 oz	37	100 g	131
Strawberry Jelly &				
Strawberries	,,	39	,,	138
Strawberry & Vanilla	,,	36	,,	127
'Kremly'				
Exotic Fruit	,,	25	,,	87
Lemon	,,	24	,,	84
Strawberry	,,	25	,,	88
'Petit Chambourcy – Aromatises'				
Apricot	,,	33	,,	118
Baked Rice & Apple	,,	39	,,	136
Chocolate Mousse	,,	52	,,	185
Egg Custard Dessert	,,	33	,,	115
Exotic Fruits	,,	35	,,	124
Strawberry	,,	35	,,	125
'Supreme Dessert'				
Chocolate & Vanilla	,,	32	,,	119
Strawberry & Vanilla	,,	38	,,	135
'Trifles'				
Black Forest Dessert	,,	36	,,	126
Fruit Cocktail	,,	31	,,	108
Raspberry	,,	33	,,	117
CHIVERS				
'Table Jellies'	1 oz	82	100 g	290

Desserts

Food	Quantities	Calories	Quantities	Calories
'Fruit For All'				
Apricot	1 oz	33	100 g	115
Blackcurrant	”	31	”	110
Morello Cherry	”	31	”	110
'Jelly Creams'				
Chocolate	”	104	”	365
Average all other flavours	”	105	”	370
CREAMOLA (dry)				
Custard Powder	1 oz	100	100 g	354
Foam Crystals (all flavours)	”	92	”	323
Rice Creamola	”	101	”	357
Steamed/Baked Pudding Mix	”	100	”	352
EDENVALE				
Cheesecake				
Blackcurrant	1 oz	50	100 g	207
Raspberry	”	55	”	194
Strawberry	”	56	”	196
Chocomousse	”	51	”	180
Creme Caramel	”	39	”	139
Creme Orange	”	40	”	141
Creme Raspberry	”	40	”	141
Fruit Softy				
Apricot	”	37	”	129
Strawberry	”	37	”	129

Food	Quantities	Calories	Quantities	Calories
Sundae				
Pear Helene	1 oz	38	100 g	132
Strawberry Champagne	,,	36	,,	128
Supreme				
Banana	,,	30	,,	105
Caramel	,,	36	,,	127
Chocolate	,,	38	,,	134
Tropical	,,	33	,,	116
Trifle				
Black Forest	,,	43	,,	152
Raspberry	,,	43	,,	153
Spanish Orange	,,	44	,,	155
Strawberry	,,	45	,,	160
FINDUS *(frozen)*				
Lemon Cream Pie	1 oz	102	100 g	358
Ripple Mousse				
Chocolate	,,	50	,,	177
Raspberry	,,	48	,,	171
Strawberry	,,	48	,,	171
HEINZ *(tinned)*				
'Sponge Puddings'				
Apple & Blackberry	1 oz	75	100 g	265
Chocolate	,,	84	,,	296
Mixed Fruit	,,	84	,,	298
Raspberry Jam	,,	81	,,	285

Desserts

Food	Quantities	Calories	Quantities	Calories
Strawberry Jam	1 oz	81	100 g	285
Treacle	”	82	”	288
HOMEPRIDE (mixes) (dry)				
Microbake Chocolate				
Pudding	1 oz	93	100 g	328
Microbake Lemon Pudding	”	91	”	319
Microbake Syrup Pudding	”	94	”	330
MARKS &SPENCER				
Pies & Tarts				
Apple Pies (6)	1 oz	92	100 g	323
Apple Puffs (6)	”	74	”	262
Apricot & Peach Pie	”	82	”	290
Deep Filled Apple Pie	”	62	”	220
Egg Custard Tarts (3)	”	76	”	267
Trellis Bramley				
Apple Tart	”	53	”	223
Cold				
Banana in Custard	”	26	”	91
Black Cherry				
Double Decker	”	35	”	124
Blackberry & Apple Fool	’	41	”	144
Blackcurrant Fruit Fool	”	47	”	165
Blackcurrant Sorbet	”	31	”	108
Caramel Delight Dessert	”	39	”	139
Charlotte Russe	”	66	”	231

Food	Quantities	Calories	Quantities	Calories
Chocolate Dairy Mousse	1 oz	24	100 g	85
Chocolate Delight Dessert	,,	39	,,	139
Chocolate Ripple	,,	36	,,	127
Chocolate Souffle	,,	47	,,	167
Creme Caramel	,,	45	,,	157
Fresh Cream Banana Trifle	,,	49	,,	174
Fresh Cream Fruit Trifle	,,	48	,,	171
Fresh Fruit Salad	,,	17	,,	60
Gooseberry Compote	,,	29	,,	101
Gooseberry Fruit Fool	'	45	,,	160
Grape & Ginger Syllabub	,,	88	,,	311
Honeydew Lemon Delight	,,	27	,,	95
Lemon Sorbet	,,	28	,,	100
Mandarin in Orange Jelly	,,	23	,,	80
Peach & Mango Delice	,,	39	,,	137
Raspberry Royale	,,	38	,,	134
Raspberry Ring	,,	39	,,	137
Rhubarb Fruit Fool	,,	38	,,	133
Rice & Apricot Purée	,,	50	,,	178
Rum Babas	,,	68	,,	240
Sherry Trifle	,,	45	,,	157
Strawberry & Guava Delice	,,	39	,,	136
Strawberry Delight Dessert	,,	33	,,	116

Desserts

Food	Quantities	Calories	Quantities	Calories
Strawberry Dairy Mousse	1 oz	22	100 g	78
Strawberry Fruit Fool	”	41	”	145
Summer Fruit Trifle	”	41	”	145
Tropical Double Decker	”	35	”	124
Hot				
Baked Jam Roll	”	111	”	390
Chocolate Pudding	”	88	”	311
Gooseberry Slice	”	90	”	318
Pancakes	”	52	”	184
Rice Pudding	”	35	”	123
Semolina Pudding	”	32	”	113
Spotted Dick	”	96	”	339
Syrup Sponge Pudding	”	106	”	375
frozen				
American Lemon Pie	”	84	”	295
Apricot Cheesecake	”	54	”	189
Blackcurrant & Apple Pie	”	77	”	271
Blackcurrant Cheesecake	”	75	”	263
Cherry & Chocolate Cheesecake	”	92	”	324
Cherry Meringue Pie	”	74	”	262
Choux Ring	”	120	”	424
Duchesse Dessert	”	64	”	224
Lemon Cream Flan	”	104	”	365
Lemon Torte	”	93	”	328
Lite Blackcurrant Cheesecake	”	52	”	185
Pecan Danish Pastry	”	104	”	368

Food	Quantities	Calories	Quantities	Calories
Raspberry & Redcurrant Cheesecake	1 oz	81	100 g	285
MR MERRY				
Carob Dessert	1 pack	82		
Custard	"	81		
Jellies	"	83		
Pineapple Dessert	"	78		
NESTLES				
Custard Powder *(dry)*	1 oz	94	100 g	330
Double Top Dessert Topping	"	50	"	178
Tip Top Dessert topping	"	31	"	110
PREWETT				
'Dessert Whip' *(dry)*				
Banana	1 oz	125	100 g	440
Carob	"	126	"	445
Strawberry	"	125	"	440
ROBERTSON				
Christmas Pudding	1 oz	92	100 g	324
ROSS *(frozen)*				
Apple Pie, Baked	1 oz	68	100 g	240
Apple & Blackberry Pie, Baked	"	68	"	240

Desserts

Food	Quantities	Calories	Quantities	Calories
'Cafe Gateaux'				
Creme Caramel	1 oz	37	100 g	130
Rich Chocolate	"	94	"	330
Strawberry	"	74	"	260
Walnut & Butterscotch	"	96	"	340
'Cheesecake'				
Strawberry	"	71	"	250
All other flavours	"	74	"	260
Dairy Cream Sponge	"	77	"	270
Devonshire Individual Trifles	"	45	"	160
'Gateaux'				
Black Forest	"	91	"	320
Black Forest Bar	"	85	"	300
Coffee Mandarin	"	88	"	310
Mandarin Cream	"	91	"	320
Mandarin Cream Bar	"	85	"	300
Strawberry & Cream	"	68	"	240
'Lighterbite Gateaux'				
Black Cherry	"	77	"	270
Triple Layer Chocolate	"	85	"	300
'Hot Puddings'				
Apple Dumplings	"	71	"	250
Apple & Blackberry Dumplings	"	71	"	250
Bread & Butter Puddings	"	73	"	150
Chocolate Fudge	"	96	"	340
Jam Roly Poly	"	105	"	370

Desserts

Food	Quantities	Calories	Quantities	Calories
Spotted Dick	1 oz	99	100 g	350
Toffee Apple Pudding	"	82	"	290
Treacle Roly Poly	"	111	"	390
ROWNTREE				
Tablet Jelly – all flavours (undiluted)	1 oz	76	100 g	268
Instant Custard Mix (dry)	"	118	"	416
ROYAL (dry)				
Cheesecake Mix	1 oz	96	100 g	337
Chocolate Mint Crunch Mix	"	97	"	343
Lemon Pie Filling Mix	"	42	"	147
Rum & Raisin Crunch Mix	"	75	"	264
Simply Topping Mix	"	51	"	179
SAFEWAY				
Dry				
Cheesecake Mix	"	84	"	296
Custard Powder	"	92	"	325
Custard, Instant	"	121	"	428
Jelly (average all flavours)	"	76	"	268
Supreme Delight				
Chocolate	"	123	"	432
average all other flavours	"	126	"	444
Fresh				
Creme Caramel	1 oz	31	100 g	110

Desserts

Food	Quantities	Calories	Quantities	Calories
Fruit Cocktail	1 oz	42	100 g	149
'Fresh Cream'				
Fruit Cocktail	"	40	"	141
Pear Trifle	"	38	"	135
Raspberry Trifle	"	36	"	127
Strawberry Trifle	"	57	"	132
Frozen				
Blackforest Gateau	"	91	"	319
Dairy Cream Sponge	"	88	"	310
Mousse, all flavours	"	45	"	160
Waffles	"	61	"	216
Tinned				
Christmas Pudding	"	91	"	319
Creamed Rice	"	25	"	88
Jam Sponge Pudding	"	102	"	359
Luxury Christmas Pudding	"	93	"	327
Rich Fruit Pudding	"	91	"	319
Semolina	"	99	"	350
Syrup Sponge Pudding	"	106	"	372
Traditional Creamed Rice	"	30	"	105
SAINSBURY				
Blackcherry Double Dessert	1 pot	47		
Chocolate Mousse	"	47		
Fresh Cream Trifle	1 oz	35	100 g	125

Food	Quantities	Calories	Quantities	Calories
ST IVEL				
'Classics'				
Lemon Pie	1 oz	72	100 g	254
Queen of Puddings	,,	49	,,	174
Syrup Sponge	,,	65	,,	229
Creme Caramel	,,	31	,,	110
'Devonshire Cheesecake'				
Blackcurrant	,,	71	,,	250
Lemon & Sultana	,,	78	,,	276
Strawberry	,,	71	,,	250
'Gateaux'				
Black Forest	,,	71	,,	250
Strawberry	,,	71	,,	250
'Snows'				
Apple	,,	36	,,	127
Raspberry	,,	46	,,	164
'Souffles'				
Chocolate	,,	54	,,	191
Lemon	,,	46	,,	163
Orange	,,	46	,,	163
'Trifles'				
Fruit Cocktail	,,	40	,,	141
Peach	,,	41	,,	145
Raspberry	,,	41	,,	144
Strawberry	,,	40	,,	143
'Wizard Mousse'				
Chocolate	,,	53	,,	186

Desserts

Food	Quantities	Calories	Quantities	Calories
Raspberry	1 oz	52	100 g	183
Strawberry	"	52	"	183
WAITROSE				
Banana Dessert	1 oz	126	100 g	444
Butterscotch Dessert	"	125	"	442
Cheesecake Mix	"	62	"	220
Chocolate Dessert	"	123	"	432
Chocolate Mousses	"	43	"	152
Chocolate Orange Dessert	"	123	"	432
Creamed Rice Pudding	"	25	"	88
Fruit Cocktail Trifle	"	38	"	134
Jelly (all flavours, undiluted)	"	77	"	272
Lemon Pie Filling Mix (dry)	"	41	"	146
Mint Chocolate Dessert	"	123	"	432
Raspberry Ripple Mousses	"	45	"	157
Raspberry Trifle	"	37	"	129
Strawberry Dessert	"	126	"	444
Strawberry & Cream Mousse (frozen)	"	42	"	149
Strawberry Ripple Mousse	"	42	"	149
Toffee & Banana Mousse	"	43	"	151
Toffee Dessert	"	126	"	444
YOUNG'S *(frozen)*				
'American Desserts'				
American Apple Pie	1 oz	65	100 g	230

Food	Quantities	Calories	Quantities	Calories
Chocolate Fudge Cake	1 oz	102	100 g	360
Deep Dish Apple				
Lattice Flan	"	68	"	240
Lemon Chiffon Cake	"	82	"	240
Mississippi Mud Pie	"	94	"	330
Passion Cake	"	118	"	415
Tennessee Grasshopper Pie	"	91	"	320
'Cheesecakes'				
Blackcurrant	"	71	"	250
Blackcurrant & Cream	"	68	"	240
Devonshire Cream	"	74	"	260
Lemon with Sultanas	"	79	"	280
Morello Cherry & Cream	"	68	"	240
Red Cherry	"	67	"	235
Strawberry	"	68	"	240
Strawberry & Cream	"	68	"	240
'Desserts'				
Apricot Brulee	"	79	"	280
Chocolate Cream Desserts	"	71	"	250
Chocolate Eclairs	"	125	"	440
Chocolate Roulade	"	105	"	370
Devonshire Creame Torte				
& Raspberries	"	77	"	270
Exotic Fruit Pavlova	"	75	"	265
Exotic Fruit Tropicana	"	75	"	265
Fruits of the Forest				
Meringue	"	79	"	280

Desserts

Food	Quantities	Calories	Quantities	Calories
Gateau Tropicana	1 oz	77	100 g	270
Hazelnut Meringue	"	136	"	480
Hazelnut Torte	"	91	"	320
Lemon Pavlova	"	84	"	295
Lemon Torte	"	82	"	290
Luxury Black Forest Gateau	"	91	"	320
Luxury Coffee Mandarin Gateau	"	78	"	275
Mandarin Charlotte Russe	"	57	"	200
Milanese Soufflé	"	70	"	245
Paris Brest with Fruit	"	91	"	320
Peach & Passion Fruit Pavlova	"	82	"	290
Peppermint Pavlova	"	108	"	380
Pineapple Pavlova	"	88	"	310
Profiteroles & Chocolate Sauce	"	94	"	330
Raspberry Charlotte Russe	"	57	"	200
Raspberry Pavlova	"	77	"	270
Raspberry & Redcurrant Brulee	"	88	"	310
Fruit Crunch	"	72	"	255
Oat Crunch	"	71	"	250
'Individual Desserts' Blackcurrant Cheesecake	each	260		

Desserts

Food	Quantities	Calories	Quantities	Calories
Brown Bread Iced Cream	1 oz	90	100 g	318
Creme Caramel	each	140		
Lemon & Sherry Syllabub	1 oz	77	100 g	271
Mixed Fruit Trifles	each	170		
Raspberry Cheesecake	"	260		
Raspberry & Redcurrant Cream Brulee	1 oz	82	100 g	290
Real Raspberry Trifles	each	170		
Real Strawberry Trifles	"	170		
Strawberry Cheesecake	"	270		

Drinks

This section is much more comprehensive than in the previous editions. However low-calorie 'diet' drinks have again been omitted, as the necessary information is listed on the packaging. Included for the first time are low-alcohol wines and beers. These products are fairly new and it is a market which is expanding rapidly. Low-calorie wines and beers are particularly useful for those who must not 'drink and drive' but it should be stressed that they are not particularly low in calories. It is therefore really better for the serious slimmer to stick to dietetic soft drinks, which are now almost indistinguishable from those containing sugar, thanks to greatly improved artificial sweeteners which no longer leave a bitter aftertaste.

Except for concentrated squashes and syrups, all amounts given are for 100 ml (3½ fl oz) as it is unlikely that anyone would drink a smaller quantity than that.

Food	Quantities	Calories	Quantities	Calories
BOOTS *(undiluted)*				
Beefy Beverage	1 oz	58	100 g	205
Drinking Chocolate, fat reduced	,,	98	,,	345
Hot Chocolate				
Instant	,,	111	,,	392
Malted	,,	112	,,	394
Malted with Honey	,,	112	,,	394
Malted	,,	102	,,	358
Night Cap	,,	102	,,	358
BOVRIL	1 tsp	10		
CADBURY *(dry)*				
Bournville Cocoa	1 portion	15	100 g	310
Bournvita	,,	20	,,	375
Chocolate Break	1 pkt	115		
Drinking Chocolate	1 portion	20		
Instant Bournvita	1 pkt	115		
CARNATION *(dry)*				
Chocolate Drink	1 oz	107	100 g	379
Chocolate Drink, sugar free	1 pkt	65		
Mellora	1 oz	40	100 g	425
HORLICKS *(dry)*				
Original	1 oz	110		
Instant	1 sachet	105		

Drinks

Food	Quantities	Calories	Quantities	Calories
Instant Chocolate Malted	1 sachet	125		
Instant Hot Chocolate	"	130		
LIFT *(dry)*				
Lemon Tea	2 tsps	35		
MARKS & SPENCER *(dry)*				
Drinking Chocolate	1 oz	105		
NESTLES				
Elevenses *(dry)*	1 tsp	5		
Milo (made with milk)	1 cup	172		
OVALTINE *(dry)*				
Chocolate Flavoured	2 tsps	10		
Choc-a-Mint	1 sachet	40		
Choc-a-Orange	"	40		
Granules	3 tsps	55		
Instant	1 sachet	120		
Instant Drinking Choc.	"	135		
OXO *(undiluted)*				
Beef Drink	1 tsp	5		
Cubes, all flavours	1 cube	15		
PREWETT				
Carob Night Time Drink *(dry)*	1 oz	97	100 g	342

Food	Quantities	Calories	Quantities	Calories
Chicory Drink	1 oz	27	100 g	97
ROWNTREE				
Cocoa *(dry)*	1 oz	87	100 g	308
SAINSBURY				
Malted Drink *(dry)*	2 tsps	55		
SAFEWAY *(dry)*				
Drinking Chocolate	1 oz	105	100 g	370
Malted Milk	"	110	"	387
WAITROSE *(dry)*				
Cocoa Powder	1 oz	93	100 g	326
Drinking Chocolate	"	112	"	395
Instant Hot Chocolate Drink	"	109	"	385
Malted Milk	"	109	"	385

Milk Shakes, Mixes & Yoghurt Drinks

CRUSHA 'Syrups'				
Banana	1 fl. oz	31	100 ml	110
Chocolate Flavour	"	46	"	162
Raspberry	"	30	"	106
Strawberry	"	30	"	106
EDENVALE				
Supershakes, all flavours	100 ml	75		

Drinks

Food	Quantities	Calories	Quantities	Calories
KELLOGG'S *(dry)*				
Two Shakes				
chocolate	1 sachet	75		
average all other flavours	"	70		
MARKS & SPENCER				
Chocolate Milkshake	100 ml	86		
Semi Skimmed				
Chocolate Drink	"	66		
Sheeps Milk Yoghurt Drink	"	100		
Strawberry Drink,				
semi-skimmed	"	57		
Yoghurt Drink,				
Strawberry/Tropical	"	73		
NESQUICK (made with milk)				
Banana & Chocolate	1 cup	184		
Raspberry	"	184		
Strawberry	"	184		
PREWETT				
Yoghurt Drink with Honey	100 ml	80		
SAINSBURY				
'Thick American Shakes' *'dry'*				
Banana/Strawberry	1 oz	80		
Chocolate	"	75		

Food	Quantities	Calories	Quantities	Calories
SPAR				
'Milk Drinks'				
Banana	100 ml	50		
Chocolate	"	60		
Strawberry	"	50		
WAITROSE				
'Milkshakes'				
Butterscotch/Fudge	100 ml	98		
Chocolate	"	73		
Strawberry	"	68		

Fruit Juices, Fruit Drinks & Squashes

Food	Quantities	Calories	Quantities	Calories
ANCHOR				
Fruit Syrups, undiluted	1 fl. oz	70		
BOOTS				
Juices				
Apple				
carbonated	100 ml	39		
English	"	47		
Pure	"	39		
Orange	"	33		
Grapefruit	"	31		
Tomato	"	16		
Squashes (concentrated)				
Blackcurrant	1 fl. oz	58	100 ml	205

Drinks

Food	Quantities	Calories	Quantities	Calories
Blackcurrant Syrup	1 fl. oz	77	100 ml	272
English Fruit Squash	"	57	"	202
Lemon Barley Drink	"	34	"	120
Lemon Honey & Ginger	"	40	"	140
Orange Barley	"	37	"	130
Tropical Fruit	"	47	"	167

BRITVIC
Juices

Food	Quantities	Calories	Quantities	Calories
Grapefruit	1 bottle	60	1 tin	90
Orange	"	50	"	75
Pineapple	"	55	"	85
Tomato or Tomato Cocktail	"	30	"	40
Tropical Fruit	"	55	"	N/A
'55'				
Apple	100 ml	44		
Grapefruit/Orange	"	50		
Pineapple	"	90		
Squashes (concentrated)				
Blackcurrant Flavour Cordial	"	35	100 ml	122
High Juice Lemon Squash	"	36	"	128
High Juice Lime Cordial	"	38	"	134
High Juice Orange Squash	"	36	"	128
Lemon Squash	"	27	"	96
Lime Flavour Cordial	"	24	"	86
Orange Squash	"	30	"	108
Peppermint Cordial	"	26	"	92

Food	Quantities	Calories	Quantities	Calories
BULMER				
Apple Juice	100 ml	37		
Grape Juice	"	43		
Kiri	"	37		
Orangina	"	37		
COPELLA				
Juice				
Apple	100 ml	40		
Blackcurrant with Apple	"	50		
Morello Cherry with Apple	"	37		
Pear with Apple	"	40		
C-VIT *(undiluted)*				
Blackcurrant Drink	1 fl. oz	60	100 ml	211
Blackcurrant & Lemon				
Barley	"	55	"	194
HEINZ				
Grapefruit	100 ml	64		
Orange	"	46		
Pineapple	"	57		
Tomato	"	22		
KELLOGG				
'Rise & Shine' *(diluted)*				
Lemon	100 ml	40		

Drinks

Food	Quantities	Calories	Quantities	Calories
All other Flavours	100 ml	44		

KIA ORA
Squashes (diluted)

Blackcurrant	100 ml	48		
Orange	”	30		
Orange & Pineapple	”	36		
Strawberry Flavour	”	38		

LIBBY
Juices

Apple 'C'	100 ml	45		
Blackcurrant 'C'	”	42		
Grapefruit Juice	”	38		
Grapefruit 'C', sweetened	”	58		
Orange Juice, sweetened	”	51		
Orange Juice, unsweetened	”	33		
Orange 'C', sweetened	”	51		
Pineapple Juice	”	53		
Tomato Juice	”	20		
Umbongo Fruit Drink	”	41		

LINDAVIA
Juices & Nectars

Apple, clear	100 ml	42		
Apple, unfiltered	”	45		

Food	Quantities	Calories	Quantities	Calories
Apricot	100 ml	60		
Blackberry	,,	29		
Blackcurrant	,,	56		
Carrot	,,	23		
Cherry	,,	55		
Grapefruit	,,	22		
Grape, Red & White	,,	63		
Orange	,,	42		
Passionfruit	,,	34		
Peach	,,	37		
Pear	,,	45		
Plum	,,	64		
Redcurrant	,,	57		
Tomato	,,	18		
Vegetable	,,	30		
MARKS & SPENCER				
Juices				
Apple & Mango	100 ml	42		
Blackcurrant Drink	,,	48		
Caribbean Drink	,,	43		
Mandarin Juice	,,	37		
Sunfruit Drink	,,	47		
'Soft Drinks & Squashes'				
Apple Sparkle	,,	46		
Blackberry & Apple Squash *(undiluted)*	1 fl. oz	63	100 ml	221

Drinks

Food	Quantities	Calories	Quantities	Calories
Blackcurrant Squash	1 fl. oz	49	100 ml	172
(undiluted)	"	49	"	172
Citro Lemon Drink	100 ml	44		
Citro Orange &				
Apricot Drink	"	35		
Lemonade	"	44		
Lemonade Plus	"	39		
Mandarin Crush	"	44		
Orange & Choc.				
Sparkling Drink	"	41		
Pear & Raspberry Squash				
(undiluted)	1 fl. oz	62	100 ml	217
Pearl	100 ml	45		
Sparkling Lemon Tea Drink	"	38		
Sunfruit Crush	"	32		
Tropical Fruit Drink				
(undiluted)	1 fl. oz	48	100 ml	169

PREWETT
Apple & Cherry	100 ml	73		
Grapefruit	"	40		
Orange, Banana & Lemon	"	36		
Orange	"	43		
Vegetable 'Country Blend'	"	27		

RIBENA
  Undiluted

Food	Quantities	Calories	Quantities	Calories
Baby Ribena	1 fl. oz	90		
Blackcurrant & Apple	,,	80		
Original	,,	80		
Ready-to-drink				
Blackcurrant & Apple/Lime	100 ml	56		
Forest Fruit Juice	,,	52		
Original	,,	60		
ROBINSON'S				
Undiluted				
'Barley Waters'				
Lemon	1 fl. oz	30	100 ml	105
Orange	,,	31	,,	110
'Whole Fruit Drinks'				
Lime Juice Cordial	,,	25	,,	90
Original Lemon	,,	39	,,	140
Original Orange	,,	44	,,	155
Special R Orange	,,	6	,,	20
Special R Orange				
& Pineapple	,,	6	,,	23
Average, all other flavours	,,	27	,,	97
'Ready Drinks'				
Apple Juice	,,	11	,,	40
Apple & Blackcurrant	,,	13	,,	45
Apple & Rasp. Juice	,,	13	,,	45
Lemon	,,	11	,,	40
Lemon Barley	,,	8	,,	30

Drinks

Food	Quantities	Calories	Quantities	Calories
Orange	1 fl. oz	10	100 ml	35
Orange, Pineapple & Lemon	"	10	"	35
Orange Barley	"	8	"	30
Original Orange	"	11	"	40
SAFEWAY				
Chilled drinks				
Blackcurrant, Lemon & Honey	100 ml	44		
English Apple Juice	"	45		
Hawaiian Drink	"	43		
Orange & Apricot Drink	"	43		
Orange Juice	"	40		
Pineapple Juice	"	43		
Tropical Fruit Drink	"	46		
Undiluted				
Apple & Rhubarb Drink	1 fl. oz	40	100 ml	140
Blackcurrant Drink	"	83	"	294
Glucose Health Drink	"	23	"	80
Lemon Drink	"	27	"	95
Lemon & Lime Drink	"	28	"	99
Lime Cordial	"	28	"	99
Orange Drink	"	27	"	94
Orange Dilute Drink	"	28	"	99
Orange & Apricot Drink	"	28	"	98

Food	Quantities	Calories	Quantities	Calories
Orange, Lemon & Pineapple Drink	1 fl. oz	29	100 ml	104
Orange & Peach Drink	"	27	"	94
Pineapple & Coconut Drink	"	25	"	90
Raspberry Drink	"	40	"	140

SPAR
Undiluted

Food	Quantities	Calories	Quantities	Calories
'High Juice' Blackcurrant	1 fl. oz	66	100 ml	229
'High Juice' Lemon/Orange	"	38	"	135
Lime Cordial	"	27	"	87
'Saver' Whole Orange	"	24	"	86
Tropical Fruit Drink	"	24	"	86
Whole Lemon Drink	"	24	"	86
Whole Orange Drink	"	24	"	86

Juices

Food	Quantities	Calories
'8' Fruit Drink	100 ml	.44
'Pure' Apple	"	42
Grapefruit	"	31
Orange	"	39
'Saver' Breakfast Orange	"	41
Sparkling Apple	"	47

VOLONTE
Juices & Nectars

Food	Quantities	Calories
Apple	100 ml	40
Grapefruit	"	36

Drinks

Food	Quantities	Calories	Quantities	Calories
Grape, Red & White	100 ml	60		
Orange	"	40		
Pineapple	"	49		
Tomato	"	16		

WAITROSE
Juice

Food	Quantities	Calories	Quantities	Calories
Apple & Cherry Cocktail	100 ml	39		
Five Fruit Juice	"	52		
Grape & Blackcurrant	"	71		
Long Life Apple & Blackcurrant	"	46		
Long Life Tropical Drink	"	43		
Natural English Apple Juice	"	43		
Orange Juice, Pure	"	35		
Orange & Apricot Drink	"	41		
Pure Apple Juice	"	43		
Pure Grapefruit Juice	"	30		
Pure Pineapple Juice	"	43		

Undiluted

Food	Quantities	Calories	Quantities	Calories
Blackcurrant Drink	1 fl. oz	65	100 ml	229
Caribbean Drink	"	24	"	85
Lemon & Lime Drink	"	24	"	85
Lime Juice Cordial	"	25	"	87
Orange Drink	"	29	"	104
Orange & Peach Drink	"	24	"	86

Food	Quantities	Calories	Quantities	Calories
Orange Squash	1 fl. oz	49	100 ml	134
Whole Lemon Drink	"	25	"	87

Sparkling Drinks

APPLETISE

APPLETISE	100 ml	44		

BARR

Iron-Bru	100 ml	40		
Lemonade	"	30		
Shandy	"	32		
Tizer	"	40		
Vimto	"	26		

BRITVIC

American Ginger Ale	100 ml	35		
Bitter Lemon Crush	"	44		
Dry Ginger Ale	"	22		
Ginger Beer	"	42		
Lime/Lemon/Orange Crush	"	50		
Tonic Water	"	31		

CANANA DRY
Carbonated

Bitter Lemon	100 ml	40		
Ginger Ale	"	38		
Indian Tonic	"	24		

Drinks

Food	Quantities	Calories	Quantities	Calories
'Rawlings'				
Passion Splitz	100 ml	45		
Apple Splitz	"	47		
CARIBA	100 ml	35		
COCA COLA	100 ml	39		
CORONA				
Banana Flavour	100 ml	24		
Berry Shandy	"	26		
Cherryade	"	26		
Coola Cola Drink	"	42		
Lemonade	"	24		
Limeade & Lager	"	32		
Traditional Lemonade	"	39		
FANTA				
Cream Soda	100 ml	28		
Ginger Beer	"	31		
Lemonade	"	24		
Limeade	"	23		
Orangeade	"	33		
Raspberryade	"	29		
Sparkling Lemon	"	35		
FERGUZADE	100 ml	93		

Food	Quantities	Calories	Quantities	Calories
HUNTS				
American Ginger Ale	100 ml	37		
Bitter Lemon	”	33		
Dry Ginger Ale	”	17		
Indian Tonic Water	”	23		
Lemonade	”	23		
KONIGSAFT				
White Grape Juice	100 ml	60		
LILT	100 ml	48		
LUCOZADE				
Glucose Drink	100 ml	73		
Lemon/Orange Barley Crush	”	72		
MANHATTAN MIXER				
Average, all flavours	100 ml	24		
MARKS & SPENCER				
Applesparkle	100 ml	.47		
Caribbean Crush	”	48		
Citro Apricot/Orange	”	35		
Citro Lemon	”	42		
Forest Fruit Crush	”	48		
Ginger Beer	”	47		
Lemonade	”	43		

Drinks

Food	Quantities	Calories	Quantities	Calories
Orange Crush	100 ml	44		
Orange Drink	"	47		
Shandy	"	23		
Sunfruit Crush	"	33		
PERRIZE	100 ml	53		
SAFEWAY				
Bitter Lemon	100 ml	55		
Cherryade	"	28		
Cherry Cola	"	45		
Cola	"	38		
Dry Ginger Ale	"	24		
Ginger Beer	"	49		
Lemonade	"	24		
Lemonade Shandy	"	13		
Limeade	"	24		
Orange	"	50		
Orange Drink	"	33		
Traditional Lemonade	"	34		
SAINSBURY				
American Ginger Ale	100 ml	13		
Bitter Lemon	"	30		
Lemonade	"	23		
Tonic Water	"	17		
All Other Flavours	"	39		

Food	Quantities	Calories	Quantities	Calories
SCHLOER				
Apple	100 ml	35		
Grape – Red & White	”	49		
SCHWEPPES				
American Ginger Ale	100 ml	22		
Bitter Lemon	”	33		
Bitter Orange	”	44		
Cascade Lemonade	”	22		
Dry Ginger Ale	”	16		
Ginger Beer	”	35		
Hi-Juice 66	”	53		
Island Fruits	”	38		
Lemonade	”	25		
Lemonade Shandy	”	26		
Limon	”	44		
Orange	”	39		
Orange & Passionfruit	”	64		
Russchian	”	22		
Strawberry	”	36		
Tonic Water	”	19		
Tropical Spring	”	30		
SEVEN UP	100 ml	38		
SPAR				
Cherryade	100 ml	.29		

Drinks

Food	Quantities	Calories	Quantities	Calories
Cola	100 ml	21		
Dandelion & Burdock	,,	19		
Keg Shandy	,,	22		
Lemonade	,,	18		
Limeade	,,	19		
Orangeade	,,	25		
'Saver' Cola	,,	24		
'Saver' Lemonade/Orange	,,	24		

STASSEN
Food	Quantities	Calories	Quantities	Calories
Apple	100 ml	45		
Apple/Apricot	,,	45		
Apple/Strawberry	,,	45		

TANGO
Food	Quantities	Calories	Quantities	Calories
Apple	100 ml	36		
Grapefruit	,,	42		
Lemon with Lime	,,	35		
Orange	,,	45		
Orange & Passionfruit	,,	44		
Orange & Pineapple	,,	44		

TOP DECK
Food	Quantities	Calories	Quantities	Calories
Lemonade & Cider	100 ml	38		
Lemonade & Lager	,,	32		
Lemonade Shandy	,,	26		

Food	Quantities	Calories	Quantities	Calories
WHITE'S				
Cherryade	100 ml	20		
Cream Soda	,,	20		
Dandelion & Burdock	,,	25		
Ginger Beer	,,	29		
Lemonade	,,	20		
Lime & Lemonade	,,	22		
Orangeade	,,	23		
Traditional Flavour Lemonade	,,	28		
ZAPPLE	100 ml	40		

Alcohol-free or virtually Alcohol-free Wines & Beers

BABYCHAM				
Dry	100 ml	57		
Sweet	,,	71		
CALVIERE	100 ml	60		
COUNTRY MANOR 'PERRY'				
Malling Grange Sparkling	100 ml	53		
Medium Dry	,,	53		
Medium Sweet	,,	63		
Pink Lady Sparkling	,,	77		
Silver Lady Sparkling	,,	70		

Drinks

Food	Quantities	Calories	Quantities	Calories
EISBERG				
Alcohol-Free Wine	100 ml	25		
GUINNESS				
Kaliber Alcohol-Free Lager	1 bottle	60		
JUNG'S				
'Alcohol-Free Wines'				
Extra Dry White	100 ml	9		
Red	"	25		
Rose	"	25		
Schloss Boosenburg	"	25		
White	"	25		
NORFOLK				
Punch	100 ml	40		
PANTHER				
Lager	100 ml	22		
PIERMONT				
Cider	100 ml	18		
SAINSBURY				
Low Alcohol Lager	1 bottle	90		
ST. CHRISTOPHER				
Low-Alcohol Lager	100 ml	14		

Fish & Shellfish

Seafood is one of the best foodstuffs there is for anybody trying to lose weight. It is, of course, preferable to eat the fresh variety but it can be noted from the following section that even the ready-prepared meals now available are usually lower in calories if made with fish. It is strongly recommended that you eat a lot of fish while on a slimming diet. There is plenty to choose from on the following pages.

Food	Quantities	Calories	Quantities	Calories
BAXTER				
Scampi with Rice				
Americaine	1 oz	31	100 g	109
Francaise	"	32	"	113
Indienne	"	32	"	113
Provencale	"	26	"	94
Thermidor	"	32	"	115
Scampi, Breaded	"	33	"	118

Fish & Shellfish

Food	Quantities	Calories	Quantities	Calories
BEJAM *(frozen)*				
'Breaded/Battered'				
Breaded Cod Fillets (fried)	1 oz	59	100 g	208
Breaded Cod Steaks	each	111		
Breaded Haddock Fillets (fried)	1 oz	63	100 g	222
Breaded Haddock Steaks	each	111		
Breaded Plaice Fillets (fried)	"	72	"	253
Breaded Scampi (fried)	1 oz	58	100 g	204
Breaded Whiting Fillets (fried)	"	61	"	215
Cod Bites	each	34		
Cod Fish Cakes	"	117		
Cod Fish Fingers	"	44		
Cod Steaks in Crispy Batter (fried)	"	248		
Haddock Steaks in Crispy Batter (fried)	each	216		
Ovenable Battered Cod Fillets (fried)	1 oz	.59	100 g	208
Supercrumb Cod Fillets	"	84	"	296
Supercrumb Plaice Fillets	"	73	"	257
Whole Boneless Breaded Plaice	"	67	"	236
Whole Plaice with Prawn and Mushroom	each	414		
'Prepared Meals'				

Food	Quantities	Calories	Quantities	Calories
Cod Bake	1 serving	297		
Cod Crumble	"	485		
Cod & Prawn Pasta	"	274		
Cod & Prawn Pie	"	408		
Haddock en Croute	"	343		
Smoked Haddock Lasagne	"	397		
BIRD'S EYE *(frozen)*				
Buttered Kipper Fillets	1 oz	55	100 g	194
Buttered Smoked Haddock	"	30	"	106
Captain's Fishburgers				
fried	each	100		
grilled or baked	"	135		
Cod Fillet Fish Fingers				
fried	"	60		
grilled	"	50		
Crunch Crumb				
fried	"	210		
grilled/baked	"	185		
Fish Cakes, Cod				
fried	"	140		
grilled	"	90		
Fish Cakes, Salmon				
fried	"	160		
grilled	"	100		
Haddock Fillet Fish Fingers				
fried	"	55		

Fish & Shellfish

Food	Quantities	Calories	Quantities	Calories
grilled	each	50		
Haddock Steaks in Crisp Crunch Crumb				
fried	”	210		
grilled	”	185		
'Menumaster Fish in Sauce'				
Cod in Butter Sauce	1 pkt	155		
Cod in Cheese Sauce	”	175		
Cod in Cream Sauce	”	125		
Cod in Mushroom Sauce	”	180		
Cod in Shrimp Flavour Sauce	”	165		
'Menumaster Fish Meals'				
Captain's Pie	10 oz	350	100 g	116
Cod Mornay	1 pkt	420		
Cod Nuggets				
grilled	1 oz	60	100 g	211
shallow fried	”	65	”	229
deep fried	”	70	”	246
Cod Steaks in Wafer Light Batter				
grilled	one	195		
shallow fried	”	220		
deep fried	”	250		
Crispy Cod Fingers (fried)	”	65		
Crispy Cod Steaks				
shallow fried	”	190		
deep fried	”	215		

Food	Quantities	Calories	Quantities	Calories
Crispy Haddock Steaks				
shallow fried	one	180		
deep fried	"	200		
Crispy Plaice Fillets				
shallow fried	1 oz	70	100 g	246
Fisherman's Choice	1 pkt	290		
Haddock Pastry Lattice	"	525		
Mariners Pasta Gratin	"	370		
Oven Crispy Cod Fish Fingers				
grilled	one	70		
shallow fried	"	80		
Oven Crispy Cod Steaks				
baked/grilled	"	215		
Oven Crispy Fish 'n Chips				
baked	1 pkt	470		
Oven Crispy Haddock Steaks				
baked/grilled	"	215		
FINDUS *(frozen)*				
Batter Crisp Cod Portions	1 oz	55	100 g	193
Batter Crisp Haddock Portion	"	64	"	224
Cod Steaks, Battered	"	49	"	173
Cod Steaks in Breadcrumbs	"	30	"	105
Cod Steak in Butter Sauce	"	23	"	81
Cod Steak in Cheese Sauce	"	25	"	89
Cod Steak in Parsley Sauce	"	18	"	65
Cod Steak in Seafood Sauce	"	20	"	71

Fish & Shellfish

Food	Quantities	Calories	Quantities	Calories
Crumb Crisp Cod Fish Fingers	1 oz	49	100 g	172
Crumb Crisp Cod Portions	″	58	″	206
Crumb Crisp Haddock Fish Fingers	″	54	″	191
Crumb Crisp Haddock Portions	″	63	″	221
Economy Fish Fingers	″	51	″	180
Fish Cakes	″	33	″	118
Haddock Steaks in Breadcrumbs	″	30	″	107
Haddock Steak in Butter Sauce	″	25	″	89
Haddock Steak in Parsley Sauce	″	19	″	66
Kipper Fillets with Butter	″	54	″	191
Prawn Curry	″	24	″	84
Smoked Haddock with Butter	″	29	″	101
JOHN WEST (tinned)				
Crab, Dressed	1 oz	38	100 g	133
Herring Fillets				
in Savoury Sauce	″	33	″	117
in Tomato Sauce	″	33	″	117
Kipper Fillets	″	64	″	227
Mackerel	″	83	″	292

Food	Quantities	Calories	Quantities	Calories
Mackerel in Brine	1 oz	57	100 g	200
Medium Red Salmon	,,	47	,,	167
Pilchards	,,	28	,,	100
Prawns	,,	24	,,	85
Pressed Cod Roes	,,	29	,,	104
Salmon				
Paté	,,	60	,,	209
Pink	,,	39	,,	138
Red	,,	60	,,	209
Sardines				
in Oil (drained)	,,	56	,,	196
in Tomato Sauce	,,	50	,,	175
Seafood Bites in Brine, drained	,,	16	,,	58
Seafood Sticks & Flakes, in Brine, drained	,,	18	,,	64
Shrimps	,,	25	,,	90
Sild				
in Oil, drained	,,	64	,,	227
in Tomato Sauce	,,	49	,,	173
Skippers, in Oil	,,	56	,,	198
Smoked Mackerel in Oil, drained	,,	89	,,	315
Tuna				
in Brine, drained	,,	25	,,	90
in Oil, drained	,,	55	,,	195

Fish & Shellfish

Food	Quantities	Calories	Quantities	Calories
MARKS & SPENCER				
Coated				
Cod Battercrisp Portions	1 oz	65	100 g	230
Cod Fillets – ovencrisp	"	69	"	243
Cod Fish Cakes	"	51	"	180
Cod Fish Fingers	"	56	"	199
Fish Fingers	"	48	"	169
Haddock in Butter	"	68	"	238
Haddock in Crispy Crumb	"	51	"	179
Haddock Kiev	"	61	"	216
Lemon Sole Breaded (frozen)	"	37	"	132
Lemon Sole Goujons	"	74	"	260
Plaice, Breaded & Boneless	"	37	"	132
Plaice Goujons	"	74	"	260
Plaice in Ovencrisp Crumb	"	74	"	260
Scots Haddock Fillets – Ovencrisp	"	64	"	225
Whiting – Ovencrisp	"	69	"	243
Smoked & Patés				
Crab Paté	"	64	"	226
Smoked Haddock Cutlets	"	27	"	96
Smoked Haddock Fillets	"	26	"	93
Kipper Fillets with Butter	"	54	"	191
Loch Fyne Kippers	"	104	"	368
Mackerel Fillets – Kippered	"	88	"	310
Smoked Mackerel Fillets	"	98	"	344
Smoked Mackerel Paté	"	90	"	318

Food	Quantities	Calories	Quantities	Calories
Smoked Rainbow Trout	1 oz	38	100 g	135
Smoked Salmon – Scottish	"	40	"	142
Smoked Salmon Paté	"	67	"	236
Prepared dishes				
Cod & Prawn Pies	"	43	"	150
Cod & Ratatouille Gratin	"	35	"	125
Cod Florentine	"	25	"	90
Cod in Butter Sauce	"	37	"	95
Cod in Parsley Sauce	"	23	"	81
Crowns of Plaice	"	32	"	114
Fish Crumble	"	38	"	133
Fisherman's Pie	"	39	"	136
Haddock Mornay	"	35	"	125
Haddock & Courgette Bake	"	26	"	92
Mariner's Bake	"	30	"	107
Moules Bonne Femme	"	38	"	133
Moules Marinière	"	24	"	85
Ocean Pie	"	30	"	107
Plaice – Filled	"	31	"	109
Salmon A La Creme	"	38	"	133

POT FISH
| Cod in Parsley | 1 pot | 210 | | |

PRINCES *(tinned)*
| Kipper Fillets | 1 tin | 590 | | |

Fish & Shellfish

Food	Quantities	Calories	Quantities	Calories
Mackerel	1 tin	435		
in Oil	"	435		
Steaks in Brine	"	255		
in Tomato Sauce	"	345		
Pilchard in Tomato Sauce	"	285		
Prawns or Shrimps	"	105		
Salmon – Pink/Red	"	155		
Sardines				
in Oil	"	415		
in Oil (drained)	"	270		
in Tomato Sauce	"	220		
Tuna				
in Oil	"	290		
ROSS *(frozen)*				
Prepared meals				
Chinese Prawns	1 oz	14	100 g	50
Cod Crumble	"	57	"	200
Cod Mornay	"	37	"	130
Cod Steaks				
in Butter Sauce	"	25	"	90
In Cheese Sauce	"	31	"	110
in Parsley Sauce	"	23	"	80
in Sweetcorn Sauce	"	23	"	80
Fish Steaks in Butter Sauce	"	25	"	90
Haddock & Prawn Crumble	"	52	"	185

Food	Quantities	Calories	Quantities	Calories
Haddock Steaks in				
Butter Sauce	1 oz	23	100 g	80
Ocean Pasta	"	34	"	120
Ocean Pie	"	34	"	120
Paella	"	35	"	125
Prawn Curry	"	20	"	70
Seafood Lasagne	"	31	"	110
Seafood Pasta	"	30	"	105
Spanish Seafood & Chicken	"	20	"	70
Smoked				
Kipper Fillets	"	60	"	210
Kipper Fillets with Butter	"	57	"	200
Kippered Mackerel Fillets	"	60	"	210
Smoked Haddock Fillets	"	23	"	80
Smoked Haddock Fillets				
with Butter	"	28	"	100
Smoked Mackerel Fillets	"	85	"	300
Smoked Whiting Fillets	"	23	"	80
Battered				
Cod Chunks	"	48	"	170
Cod Fillet Chip Shop	"	54	"	190
Crispy Cod	"	48	"	170
Crispy Haddock	"	48	"	170
Haddock Fillet Chip Shop	"	51	"	180
Jumbo Cod Fingers	"	54	"	190
Oven Cod	"	57	"	200

Fish & Shellfish

Food	Quantities	Calories	Quantities	Calories
Breaded				
Cod Fillets	1 oz	48	100 g	170
Cod Steaks	"	48	"	170
Fish Cakes – Traditional	"	34	"	120
Fish Fingers	"	54	"	190
Haddock Fillets	"	54	"	190
Haddock Steaks	"	54	"	190
SAFEWAY				
Frozen				
Cod in Batter	1 oz	57	100 g	200
Cod in Breadcrumbs	"	60	"	212
Cod in Butter Sauce	"	26	"	90
Cod in Parsley Sauce	"	23	"	80
Cod Fillets in Breadcrumbs	"	45	"	160
Cod Fish Fingers	"	52	"	184
Fish Cakes	"	34	"	121
Fish Fingers	"	52	"	184
Haddock in Batter	"	57	"	200
Haddock in Breadcrumbs	"	60	"	211
Haddock Fillets in Breadcrumbs	"	43	"	153
Plaice Fillets in Breadcrumbs	"	48	"	171
Tinned				
Sardines in Oil	"	95	"	334
Sardines in Tomato Sauce	"	50	"	177
Tuna in Brine	"	28	"	97

Food	Quantities	Calories	Quantities	Calories
Tuna in Oil	1 oz	67	100 g	237
Chilled				
Smoked Mackerel Fillets				
with Garlic	"	63	"	222
Honey & Peaches	"	55	"	195
Lemon & Tarragon	"	63	"	222
Mixed Herbs	"	63	"	222
Pineapple & Olives				
(Carribean)	"	56	"	196
SAINSBURY				
Frozen				
Cod & Broccoli Pie	1 pack	365	100 g	100
Cod & Prawn Casserole	"	180	"	50
Cod & Prawn Pie with Grapes	"	445	"	160
Cod & Vegetable Pasta	"	275	"	90
Cod in Batter, fried	"	60	"	211
Cod in Breadcrumbs	"	59	"	208
Cod in Butter Sauce	"	32	"	113
Fish Cakes				
fried	each	150		
grilled	"	90		
Fish Fingers				
fried	"	65		
grilled	"	50		
Plaice stuffed with Broccoli/Cheese				
deep fried	one	410		

Fish & Shellfish

Food	Quantities	Calories	Quantities	Calories
Salmon/Asparagus en croute	1 serving	415	100 g	245
Scampi in Breadcrumbs	1 oz	90		
Seafood Fettuccine	1 serving	650		
Tinned				
Mackerel Fillet				
in Brine	1 oz	54	100 g	190
in oil	”	84	”	295
in tomato	”	52	”	185
Salmon				
pink	”	38	”	135
medium red	”	41	”	145
red	”	47	”	165
Sardines				
in oil	”	60	”	210
in tomato sauce	”	50	”	175
Tuna				
in brine	”	34	”	120
in veg oil	”	45	”	160
skipjack in oil	”	45	”	160
SPAR				
Frozen				
Cod Fish Fingers	1 oz	52	10 oz	183
Cod Steak in Butter Sauce	”	23	”	81
Cod Steak in Parsley Sauce	”	23	”	81

Food	Quantities	Calories	Quantities	Calories
WAITROSE				
Frozen				
Breaded Cod Fillets	1 oz	.31	100 g	110
Breaded Lemon Sole Goujons	,,	43	,,	150
Breaded Plaice Fillets	,,	31	,,	110
Haddock Goujons	,,	40	,,	140
Kippers, Boned	,,	54	,,	190
Kipper Cutlets	,,	54	,,	190
Kipper Fillets	,,	54	,,	190
Kippers, Whole	,,	43	,,	152
Plaice in Butter Sauce	,,	57	,,	200
Plaice in a Mornay Sauce	,,	54	,,	190
Prawns, cooked & peeled	,,	30	,,	107
Smoked Cod Fillets	,,	29	,,	101
Smoked Haddock Fillets	,,	23	,,	80
Patés				
Crab	,,	56	,,	196
Scottish Smoked Salmon	,,	58	,,	204
Smoked Mackerel	,,	62	,,	220
Smoked Salmon	,,	76	,,	267
Smoked Trout	,,	75	,,	264
Prepared meals				
Cod & Broccoli Mornay	,,	29	,,	102
Fisherman's Pie	,,	37	,,	130
Smoked Haddock Savoury Bake	,,	46	,,	163

Fish & Shellfish

Food	Quantities	Calories	Quantities	Calories
Smoked, fresh				
Cod Fillets	1 oz	29	100 g	101
Finnan Haddock	,,	29	,,	101
Haddock Fillets	,,	28	,,	99
Kippers	,,	58	,,	205
Mackerel Fillets	,,	73	,,	256
Mackerel Fillets with crushed Peppercorns	,,	73	,,	256
Tinned				
Pink Salmon	,,	40	,,	141
Red Sockeye Salmon	,,	46	,,	163
Sardines in Oil	,,	56	,,	198
Sardines in Tomato	,,	50	,,	177
Skipjack Tuna in Brine	,,	33	,,	117
Skipjack Tuna in Oil	,,	75	,,	264
YOUNG'S				
Chilled				
Cod & Parsley Croquettes	1 oz	.54	100 g	192
Filled Plaice with Butter Sauce	,,	45	,,	158
Filled Plaice with Mornay Sauce	,,	45	,,	158
Fresh Cod in Breadcrumbs	,,	51	,,	179
Fresh Cod Fishcakes	,,	60	,,	213
Fresh Fish Kebabs	,,	16	,,	56

Fish & Shellfish

Food	Quantities	Calories	Quantities	Calories
Fresh Haddock in Breadcrumbs	1 oz	55	100 g	193
Fresh Plaice in Breadcrumbs	,,	71	,,	249
Fresh Smoked Cod Fillets	,,	22	,,	78
Fresh Smoked Haddock Cutlets	,,	25	,,	87
Fresh Smoked Haddock Fillets	,,	22	,,	78
Kippers	,,	60	,,	213
Kipper Cutlets	,,	60	,,	213
Kippered Mackerel	,,	92	,,	323
Lemon Sole Fillets	,,	23	,,	82
Lemon Sole Goujons	,,	63	,,	223
Sea Scallops in Breadcrumbs	,,	48	,,	168
Seafood Sticks	,,	24	,,	85
Sea Scallops	,,	26	,,	93
Smoked Fish Kebabs	,,	38	,,	134
Smoked Haddock Croquettes	,,	53	,,	188
Smoked Haddock Fillets	,,	25	,,	87
Whole Scampi Tails in Breadcrumbs	,,	58	,,	203
Prepared meals				
Cod & Prawn Pies	,,	55	,,	195
Crab Thermidor	,,	37	,,	130
Garlic Prawns	,,	21	,,	75
Lemon Sole Bonne Femme	,,	24	,,	85
Oriental Prawns	,,	31	,,	110

Fish & Shellfish

Food	Quantities	Calories	Quantities	Calories
Prawn Quiche	1 oz	68	100 g	240
Salmon En Croute	,,	77	,,	270
Scampi Provençale	,,	18	,,	65
Seafood Pasta	,,	34	,,	120
Seafood Lasagne	,,	31	,,	110
Trout Almande	,,	45	,,	160
Trout Veronique	,,	37	,,	130
Frozen				
Cod & Parsley Croquettes	,,	54	,,	192
Filled Plaice with Butter Sauce	,,	45	,,	158
Filled Plaice with Mornay Sauce	,,	45	,,	158
Fresh Fish Kebabs	,,	16	,,	56
Fresh Haddock in Breadcrumbs	,,	55	,,	193
Fresh Plaice in Breadcrumbs	,,	55	,,	193
Fresh Smoked Cod Fillets	,,	22	,,	78
Fresh Smoked Haddock Cutlets	,,	25	,,	87
Fresh Smoked Haddock Fillets	,,	22	,,	78
Haddock Dippers	,,	55	,,	193
Kippers	,,	60	,,	213
Kippered Mackerel	,,	92	,,	323
Lemon Sole Fillets	,,	23	,,	82

Food	Quantities	Calories	Quantities	Calories
Lemon Sole Goujons	1 oz	63	100 g	223
Peppered Mackerel	,,	95	,,	333
Sea Scallops in Breadcrumbs	,,	48	,,	168
Seafood Sticks	,,	24	,,	85
Sea Scallops	,,	26	,,	93
Smoked Fish Kebabs	,,	38	,,	134
Smoked Haddock Croquettes	,,	53	,,	188
Smoked Pacific Salmon	,,	40	,,	142
Smoked Scotch Salmon	,,	40	,,	142
Whole Scampi Tails in Breadcrumbs	,,	58	,,	203
Prepared Meals				
Cod & Prawn Pies	each	406	100 g	195
Crab Thermidor	1 pack	410	100 g	130
Garlic Prawns	,,	179	,,	75
Lemon Sole Bonne Femme	,,	155	,,	85
Oriental Prawns	,,	262	,,	110
Prawn Quiche	whole quiche	857	,,	240
Salmon en Croute	each	425	,,	270
Scampi Provencale	1 pack	120	,,	65
Seafood Pasta	,,	607	,,	120
Seafood Lasagne	,,	589	,,	110
Trout Almande	,,	605	,,	160
Trout Veronqique	,,	232	,,	130

Fruit

Fruit which has been tinned in juice rather than syrup is now much more widely available and is a boon to slimmers. If you must eat fruit tinned in syrup then be sure and drain all the syrup carefully as that is the fattening part. All the fruits listed below are in *syrup* unless otherwise indicated. It can be seen that the calorific content does not vary much from brand to brand. In the case of dried fruit there is no difference, so these have not been included in this book. Check in any calorie-counter for their calorific content.

Food	Quantities	Calories	Quantities	Calories
HARTLEY				
Tinned				
Blackcurrants	1 oz	17	100 g	60
Damsons	"	24	"	85
Gooseberries	"	20	"	70
Prunes	"	27	"	95

Food	Quantities	Calories	Quantities	Calories
Raspberries	1 oz	20	100 g	70
Strawberries	”	33	”	115

LIBBY
Tinned

Apricots	1 oz	20	100 g	69
Chunky Mixed Fruits				
(in juice)	”	15	”	52
Fruit Cocktail	”	22	”	79
Grapefruit Segments				
(in juice)	”	8	”	30
Peaches	”	20	”	69
Peach Halves	”	20	”	69
Peach Halves in Natural Juice	”	13	”	47
Peach Slices in Natural Juice	”	14	”	49
Pear Halves in Natural Juice	”	14	”	49
Pineapple Slices	”	16	”	57
Pineapple Slices in Natural				
Juice	”	15	”	54
Pineapple Tidbits	”	16	”	58

SAFEWAY
Tinned

Fruit Cocktail	1 oz	20	100 g	69
Peach Halves/Slices	”	19	”	68
Peaches & Pears	”	19	”	68
Pear Halves	”	22	”	77

Fruit

Food	Quantities	Calories	Quantities	Calories
Pear Quarters	1 oz	20	100 g	69
Pear Halves (in Juice)	,,	14	,,	50
Pineapple (in Juice)	,,	14	,,	50
Spanish Mandarins	,,	16	,,	56
Strawberries	,,	20	,,	69
SAINSBURY				
Apricot Halves in Juice	1 oz	9	100 g	32
Apricot Halves	,,	17	,,	60
Blackberries in Juice	,,	10	,,	35
Blackcurrants in Fruit Juice	,,	11	,,	40
Fruit Cocktail in Juice	,,	11	,,	39
Fruit Cocktail	,,	21	,,	74
Gooseberries	,,	21	,,	74
Grapefruit Segments in Juice	,,	11	,,	40
Grapefruit Segments	,,	21	,,	74
Mandarin Oranges	,,	19	,,	67
Peaches	,,	19	,,	67
Peach Slices in Juice	,,	10	,,	35
Pears	,,	19	,,	67
Pineapple	,,	19	,,	67
Plums	,,	31	,,	109
Raspberries	,,	25	,,	88
Raspberries in Juice	,,	9	,,	32
Rhubarb	,,	21	,,	74
Satsuma Segments in Juice	,,	11	,,	39

Food	Quantities	Calories	Quantities	Calories
WAITROSE				
Apricot Halves in Juice	1 oz	11	100 g	38
Apricot Halves	"	25	"	89
Fruit Cocktail in Apple Juice	"	14	"	50
Fruit Cocktail	"	27	"	95
Fruit Salad	"	18	"	62
Grapefruit Segments in Juice	"	10	"	36
Grapefruit Segments	"	18	"	62
Mandarin Oranges	"	19	"	67
Mandarin Oranges in Juice	"	13	"	45
Peach Slices in Juice	"	10	"	35
Peach Slices	"	21	"	75
Pear Quarters in Juice	"	14	"	50
Pear Quarters	"	20	"	71
Pineapple Pieces in Juice	"	17	"	59
Pineapple Pieces	"	21	"	76
Pie Fillings				
Apple Fruit Filling	"	21	"	76
Apple & Blackberry Fruit Filling	"	18	"	62
Apricot Fruit Filling	"	18	"	64
Black Cherry Fruit Filling	"	20	"	70
Blackcurrant Fruit Filling	"	22	"	78
Prunes	"	34	"	120

Health Bars

There are many more of these delicious snacks around today and they are to be found in sweet shops and grocery stores as well as health food shops. They are unfortunately usually as high in calories as ordinary confectionary but they do also supply you with nutritionally valuable ingredients. So if you feel like indulging in something sweet try to pick something from this section.

Food	Quantities	Calories	Quantities	Calories
ALLINSON				
Carobran	1 bar	135	100 g	385
Carob Coated Sesame Crunch	"	117	"	469
Carob Crunch	"	150	"	471
'Fruit Bars				
Banana	"	88	"	251
Fruit & Nut	"	112	"	320
Muesli	"	108	"	308
Fruit Crunch	"	119	"	425

Food	Quantities	Calories	Quantities	Calories
Nut Crunch	1 bar	130	100 g	464
AVALANCHE				
Citrus Bar	1 bar	193	100 g	483
Fruit & Nut Bar	”	191	”	478
BOOTS				
Coconut Crunch	1 oz	128	100 g	452
Date & Museli	”	92	”	324
Fruit & Nut with Honey	”	127	”	447
Fruit Muesli	”	107	”	377
Ginger & Pear	”	98	”	344
Honey Crunch	”	123	”	432
Natural Poppy Seed	”	125	”	439
Natural Sesame Seed	”	132	”	464
Natural Sunflower	”	132	”	464
Oat & Honey Crunch	”	123	”	432
Swiss Style Muesli	”	99	”	350
CLUSTER				
Apple & Hazelnut	1 oz	108	100 g	381
Apricot & Chocolate Chip	”	109	”	384
Hazelnut & Raisin	”	119	”	418
Peanut & Almond	”	131	”	463
GRANOSE 'Bars				
Apricot Date	30 g bar	85		

Health Bars

Food	Quantities	Calories	Quantities	Calories
Blackberry	50 g bar	188		
Cherry	"	187		
Carob-Coated Fruit	35 g bar	145		
Carob-Coated Muesli	"	145		
Carob-Coated Pineapple	"	145		
Date	25 g bar	87		
Date and Apricot	"	85		
Date and Coconut	"	102		
Date and Fig	"	80		
Date and Nut	"	95		
Date and Sesame	"	92		
Fig and Prune	25 g bar	77		
Fig and Raisin	"	85		
Ginger Pear	30 g bar	110		
Hazelnut	50 g bar	238		
Lemon	"	184		
Mixed Fruit	"	192		
Orange	"	188		
Rosehip	"	191		
Strawberry	"	187		
'Soft Muesli'				
Apple	25 g bar	104		
Chocolate Chip	"	121		
Hazelnuts	"	119		
Hazelnut and Almond	"	115		
HOLLY MILLS 'Bars'				
Apple & Cardamon	1 bar	170	100 g	424

Food	Quantities	Calories	Quantities	Calories
Apple & Hazelnut	1 bar	147	100 g	490
Apricot and Almond	”	156	”	390
Apricot Honey	”	83	”	277
Apricot Malt	”	79	”	263
Banana Fruit	”	93	”	345
Banana Munch	”	142	”	475
Carob Chip	”	147	”	490
Carob-coated	”	137	”	390
'Castaway' Carob Topped				
Apple & Hazelnut	”	200	”	500
Banana	”	212	”	530
Crunchy	”	197	”	492
Fibre-Time Snack	”	147	”	387
Oat Apple & Raisin	”	194	”	441
Oat Apricot & Almond	”	203	”	461
Oat & Sesame Seed	”	135	”	453
Oat & Sunflower Seed	”	136	”	455
Protein	”	183	”	416
Roasted Peanut	”	156	”	520
'Square Snacks'				
Crunchy Oat & Nut	”	187	”	407
Muesli	”	216	”	432
Oat, Fruit & Nut	”	174	”	414
JORDANS				
'Original Crunchy Bars'				
Apple & Bran	1 bar	131	100 g	394
Coconut & Honey	”	139	”	416

Health Bars

Food	Quantities	Calories	Quantities	Calories
Honey & Almonds	1 bar	137	100 g	412
Orange & Carob	"	140	"	420
KALIBU				
Carob Chips	1 oz	139	100 g	493
'Carob Coated'				
Peanuts	"	144	"	510
Peanuts & Raisins	"	131	"	465
Raisins	"	122	"	431
Crunchy Bran & Raisin	"	122	"	432
Fruit & Nut Kalibu				
No Added Sugar	"	136	"	483
Fruit & Nut Kalibu				
With Raw Sugar	"	131	"	463
Orange Kalibu				
No Added Sugar	"	139	"	493
Orange Kalibu				
With Raw Sugar	"	139	"	493
Peanut Butters	"	182	"	646
Peanut Kalibu				
with No Added Sugar	"	143	"	507
Peppermint Kalibu				
No Added Sugar	"	139	"	493
Plain Kalibu				
No Added Sugar	"	139	"	493
Plain Kalibu				
with Raw Sugar	"	139	"	493

Food	Quantities	Calories	Quantities	Calories
'Snack Bars'				
Banana Chew	1 oz	92	100 g	326
Cherry Chew	”	115	”	409
Fruit Bar	”	95	”	338
Ginger Fudge	”	117	”	414
Marzipan	”	123	”	435
Raisin	”	96	”	339
Raspberry Yoghurt	”	116	”	411
'Yogurt Break'				
All flavours	”	149	”	526
'Yogurt Coated'				
Peanuts	”	154	”	546
Peanuts & Raisins	”	143	”	508
Raisins	”	125	”	442
PREWETT				
Apple & Date	1 bar	108	100 g	257
Apple & Ginger	”	140	”	333
Banana	”	105	”	251
'Carob-Coated'				
Banana	”	128	”	305
Date & Fig	”	142	”	337
Muesli	”	148	”	353
Orange & Sultana	”	156	”	372
Date & Fig	”	123	”	294
Fruit & Bran	”	125	”	297
Fruit & Nut	”	134	”	320

Health Bars

Food	Quantities	Calories	Quantities	Calories
Muesli	1 bar	129	100 g	308
Orange & Sultana	"	143	"	340
QUAKER				
'Harvest Crunch Bars'				
Almond	1 bar	85	100 g	470
Choc. Chip	"	113	"	445
Choc. & Hazelnut	"	81	"	450
Fruit & Nut	"	108	"	425
Peanut	"	83	"	460
Raisin	"	79	"	440

Ice Cream

Ice cream is actually not as high in calories as you might expect, as long as you avoid the varieties made with real cream. It can quickly be seen that there is a big difference in the calorific content of various types, even those from the same company. For example, Wall's plain vanilla has 176 calories per 100 grams while the same company's Mint Chocolate Croccante has 229. Quite a difference! So be careful to choose one of the types with less calories if you are on a strict diet. There are certainly plenty to choose from here.

Food	Quantities	Calories	Quantities	Calories
BEJAM *(frozen)*				
Black Cherry & Kirsch	1 oz	48	100 g	169
Cassata	"	47	"	165
Choc 'n' Nut Choc Ices	each	119		
Choc 'n' Nut	1 oz	64	100 g	225

Ice Cream

Food	Quantities	Calories	Quantities	Calories
Choc 'n' Nut Cornets	each	258		
Choc 'n' Nut Split Lollies	"	158		
Choc 'n' Nut Sundae	"	177		
Choc Orange with Contreau	1 oz	48	100 g	169
Chocolate/Orange Bombe	each	177		
Coffee	1 oz	47	100 g	165
Crunchy Toffee	"	57	"	201
Dark Choc Ices	each	115		
Dark Mint Choc Ices	"	115		
Economy Vanilla	1 oz	35	100 g	123
Golden Choc Ices	each	115		
Ice Cream Roll	1/6 roll	82		
Mint Choc Chip	1 oz	48	100 g	169
Neapolitan	"	45	"	165
Neapolitan Chequers	"	46	"	162
Neapolitan Choc Ices	each	119		
Knickerbocker Glory	"	272		
Orange Lollies	"	20		
Passion Fruit & Peach	1 oz	51	100 g	179
Peach Melba Sundae	each	177		
Pineapple & Coconut	1 oz	47	100 g	165
Raspberry Ripple	"	48	"	169
Sno Ice Lolly	each	83		
Strawberry/Vanilla Bombes	"	193		
Sugar-Free Orange Lolly	"	35		
White Vanilla	1 oz	45	100 g	158

Food	Quantities	Calories	Quantities	Calories
BERTORELLI				
Bombe – Dairy Cassata	each	614	100 g	215
Chocolate – Dairy	1 oz	60	100 g	211
Chocolate Menthe	”	66	”	233
Coffee	”	56	”	196
Lemon Water Ice	”	31	”	109
Mela Menthe	each	213	”	306
Mela Parisienne	”	211	”	302
Mela Stragata	”	208	”	298
Orange Water Ice	1 oz	31	”	110
Praline – Dairy	”	60	”	210
Raspberry Water Ice	”	29	”	101
Strawberry – Dairy	”	50	”	176
Surprise				
Lemon	each	158	”	225
Orange		176	”	220
Vanilla – Dairy		57	”	202
LOSELEY				
Ice Cream				
Acacia Honey & Ginger	1 oz	53	100 g	188
Brazilian Mocha	”	60	”	212
Montezuma Chocolate	”	47	”	167
Old Fashioned Vanilla	”	57	”	202
Passion Fruit I-N-Cream	”	19	”	66
Sovereign Strawberry	”	45	”	160
Woodland Hazel	”	57	”	200

Ice Cream

Food	Quantities	Calories	Quantities	Calories
Sorbet	1 oz	22	100 g	79
Apricot	"	22	"	79
Blackcurrant	"	20	"	69
Lemon	"	19	"	67
Pineapple	"	21	"	74
LYONS MAID				
'Cutting Bricks'				
Chocolate Ripple	1 oz	51	100 g	181
Neapolitan	"	51	"	179
Peach Melba	"	50	"	177
Raspberry Ripple	"	49	"	173
Vanilla	"	52	"	182
Weight Watchers	"	27	"	97
'Family Bricks'				
Chocolate/Banana	"	51	"	181
Cornish Dairy	"	57	"	202
Fruit Harvest				
Pineapple	"	43	"	150
Raspberry	"	49	"	174
Neopolitan	"	51	"	179
Vanilla	"	52	"	182
Weight Watchers	"	27	"	97
'Gold Seal'				
Caramel Toffee	"	60	"	210
Chocolate Coconut Flake	"	52	"	183
Chocolate Swirl	"	54	"	192

Food	Quantities	Calories	Quantities	Calories
Mint Chocolate Chip	1 oz	56	100 g	196
Rum & Raisin	"	52	"	184
Vanilla Chocolate Flake	"	62	"	219
'Individual Lines'				
Barmy Banana	each	78		
Big Squeeze	"	109		
Chockle	"	72		
Cocktail				
Blue Hawaiian	"	34		
Brandy Alexander	"	81		
Pina Colada	"	60		
MARKS & SPENCER				
Luxury Dairy Vanilla	1 oz	75	100 g	263
Orange Juice Bars	"	25	"	90
Raspberry Ripple Dairy	"	49	"	174
Rum & Raisin	"	57	"	200
Soft Scoop Vanilla	"	52	"	183
Soft Scoop Vanilla, non-dairy	"	48	"	170
Vanilla, dairy	"	50	"	178
Walnut Supreme	"	68	"	239
ROSS				
Chocolate	1 oz	51	100 g	180
Chocolate Ripple	"	51	"	180
Dairy Cornish	"	45	"	160
Raspberry Ripple	"	48	"	170

Ice Cream

Food	Quantities	Calories	Quantities	Calories
Strawberry	1 oz	48	100 g	170
Vanilla	"	48	"	170
Vanilla Choc Ices	each	130	"	290
SAFEWAY				
Banana Soft Scoop	1 oz	48	100 g	169
Chocolate Soft Scoop	"	47	"	167
Cornish Cutting Brick	"	48	"	169
Cornish Vanilla Family Brick	"	48	"	169
Economy Ice Cream	"	51	"	179
Ice Cream Roll	"	50	"	178
'Luxury'				
Apple Pie	"	65	"	228
Country Strawberry Dairy	"	62	"	218
Egg Nog & Raisin Dairy	"	65	"	229
Georgia Pecan Pie	"	68	"	239
Jaffa Orange	"	63	"	221
Maple & Walnut	"	66	"	233
Mocha Almond	"	73	"	259
Pina Colada Dairy	"	63	"	221
Praline & Toffee Dairy	"	65	"	230
Tin Roof Dairy	"	69	"	242
Vanilla Dairy	"	64	"	225
Orange Ice Lollies	"	12	"	42
Raspberry Ripple				
Cutting Brick	"	46	"	164

Food	Quantities	Calories	Quantities	Calories
Raspberry Ripple Family Brick	1 oz	46	100 g	164
Raspberry Ripple Soft Scoop	”	49	”	172
Strawberry Cutting Brick	”	50	”	182
Vanilla Choc Ices	”	75	”	263
Vanilla Cutting Brick	”	52	”	182
Vanilla Family Brick	”	52	”	182
Vanilla Soft Scoop	”	48	”	169

SAINSBURY

Food	Quantities	Calories	Quantities	Calories
Blackcurrant Fruit Dairy	1 oz	54	100 g	190
Chocolate Ribonette Dairy	”	54	”	190
Natural Strawberry	”	54	”	190
Natural Vanilla	”	54	”	190
Vanilla	”	54	”	190

WAITROSE

'American Style'

Food	Quantities	Calories	Quantities	Calories
Chocolate Chip	1 oz	55	100 g	194
Chocolate Orange	”	55	”	195
Mint Chocolate Chip	”	56	”	199
Strawberry & Cream	”	50	”	178
Blackcurrant Sorbet	”	37	”	132
Choc Chip Choc Ices (10)	”	88	”	309
Choc Ices, Dark & Milk	”	82	”	290
Chocolate Ice Cream	”	52		185

page 169

Ice Cream

Food	Quantities	Calories	Quantities	Calories
Coffee	1 oz	44	100 g	154
Cornish Dairy	”	49	”	173
Lemon Sorbet	”	32	”	114
Neopolitan	”	45	”	157
Passion Fruit Sorbet	”	35	”	125
Pineapple & Coconut				
Choc Ices (10)	”	82	”	288
Raspberry Ripple	”	55	”	193
Soft Vanilla	”	44	”	155
Strawberry	’	54	”	189
Vanilla	”	45	”	158
Vanilla Slicing Pack	”	48	”	171
WALL'S				
'Alpine'				
Chocolate	1 oz	59	100 g	209
Lemon Sorbet	”	40	”	142
Orange Sorbet	”	40	”	142
Strawberry	”	57	”	200
Vanilla	”	59	”	209
'Carte D'Or'				
Blackcurrant Sorbet	”	37	”	130
Cherry Kirsch	”	34	”	121
Chocolate	”	36	”	126
Coffee	”	33	”	115
Lemon Sorbet	”	37	”	130
Orange Sorbet	”	37	”	130

Food	Quantities	Calories	Quantities	Calories
Strawberry	1 oz	34	100 g	120
Vanilla	"	35	"	123
Walnut	"	39	"	138
'Family Bricks, Packs'				
Bananarama	"	45	"	158
Blue Ribbon Vanilla	1 brick	460		
Chocl 'n' Nut Slice	"	430		
Cornish Vanilla	1 oz	52	"	183
Cream of Cornish	"	52	"	183
Golden Vanilla	"	50	"	176
Neapolitan	"	50	"	176
Pinacolada	"	42	"	148
Raspberry Ripple	"	50	"	176
Rum and Raisin	"	52	"	183
Strawberry Ripple	"	52	"	183
'Italiano'				
Choc & Nut Capri	"	60	"	211
Fruits of the Forest	"	45	"	158
Mint Choc Croccante	"	65	"	229
Strawberry Rosama	"	45	"	158
Toffee Fudge Caramella	"	57	"	201
Tutti Frutti Classico	"	52	"	183
'Soft Scoop'				
Blue Ribbon Vanilla	"	50	"	176
Golden Vanilla	"	52	"	183
Raspberry Ripple	"	50	"	176
Rum & Raisin	"	52	"	183

Ice Cream

Food	Quantities	Calories	Quantities	Calories
'Specials				
Cassata Denise Log	each	585		
Choc 'n' Hazelnut Log	"	700		
Harlequin – chocolate/				
strawberry	"	540		
Mint Whip	"	200		
Viennetta	"	815		
'Twinpack'				
Bananarama	1 oz	45	100 g	158
Hawaiian Punch	"	47	"	165
Strawberry & Chocolate	"	52	"	183
Strawberry & Vanilla	"	50	"	176
Summer Days	"	45	"	158
'In Hand Lines'				
B.A.	each	45		
Banana & Choc. Megabyte	"	120		
Blue Ribbon Vanilla Tub	"	130		
Choc 'n' Nut Italiano	"	175		
Choc Mint Cup Italiano	"	170		
Choco Rico Premium Cone	"	240		
Cornetto				
Choc'n'Nut	"	205		
Neapolitan	"	195		
Strawberry	"	190		
Tuttie Frutti	"	230		
Cornish Ice Cream Bar	"	90		
Dark & Golden Choc Bars	"	135		

Food	Quantities	Calories	Quantities	Calories
Double Choc Bar	each	165		
Fame	"	100		
Fat Frog	"	50		
Feast	"	260		
Florida Orange Mini Fruit	"	30		
Funny Faces	"	.75		
Funny Feet	"	85		
Golden Vanilla Choc Bar	"	135		
Googles Bar	"	100		
Ice Cream Bar				
Dairy Vanilla	"	90		
Golden Vanilla	"	85		
Jelly Jumbo	"	105		
Mini Milk				
Strawberry	"	40		
Vanilla	"	85		
Nutty Choc Bar	"	180		
Orange Fruttie	"	80		
Pineapple Split	"	85		
Raspberry Crush Cup Italiano	each	120		
Raspberry/Strawberry Cup				
Italiano	"	110		
Romero	"	170		
Screwball – 2 ball	"	115		
Sparkles, average all flavours	"	30		
Starship 4	"	35		
Strawberry Individual Slice	"	60		

Ice Cream

Food	Quantities	Calories	Quantities	Calories
Strawberry Split	each	80		
Toffee & Choc. Megabyte	"	120		
Tongue Twister	"	85		
Tom & Jerry	"	55		
Tropical Fruit Water Ice	"	55		
Vanilla Individual Slice	"	65		

Jam, Marmalade, Honey, Spreads

New since the last edition of this book are the excellent 'fruit spreads' which are sugar-free and therefore lower in calories. These should be used in preference to jams but they do have the one disadvantage that they do not keep indefinitely and one is therefore inclined to use more to avoid waste! Since the number of calories in different flavours of jam varies hardly at all they have not been listed separately.

Food	Quantities	Calories	Quantities	Calories
BAXTER				
Jams – average all flavours	1 oz	68	100 g	242
Wild Bramble Jelly	"	73	"	259
'Marmalade'				
'Castle' Orange	"	71	"	250
Fine Shred Lemon	"	72	"	253
Lime	"	72	"	253
Fine Shred Orange	"	71	"	250

Jam, Marmalade, Honey, Spreads

Food	Quantities	Calories	Quantities	Calories
Grapefruit	1 oz	70	100 g	247
Scotch Orange	"	69	"	246
Three Fruits	"	70	"	247
'Vintage' Orange	"	72	"	254
CADBURY				
Chocolate Spread	1 portion	45	100 g	315
Hazelnut Choc. Spread	"	85	"	570
BOOTS				
Honey	1 oz	82	100 g	288
Peanut Butter				
Smooth & Crunchy	"	172	"	605
CHIVERS				
Extra	1 portion	40	100 g	255
Lemon Curd	"	45	"	285
Marmalades	"	40	"	255
CROSSE & BLACKWELL				
Redcurrant Jelly	1 oz	73	100 g	259
FERRERO				
Nutella	1 oz	149	100 g	525
GALES				
Honey, Set & Clear	1 oz	87	100 g	310

Jam, Marmalade, Honey, Spreads

Food	Quantities	Calories	Quantities	Calories
Lemon Curd	1 oz	79	100 g	280
Peanut Butter				
Smooth & Crunchy	,,	165	,,	586
HARTLEYS				
Jelly Jams	1 oz	40	100 g	260
Lemon Cheese	,,	45	,,	295
Marmalade	,,	40	,,	255
Mincemeat	,,	45	,,	285
Pure Fruit Jams	,,	40	,,	255
MARKS & SPENCER				
Honey – average all flavours	1 oz	82	100 g	290
Jam – average all flavours	,,	68	,,	240
MOORHOUSE				
Jams	1 oz	40	100 g	255
Lemon Cheese	,,	45	,,	295
Lemon Curd	,,	45	,,	285
Marmalade	,,	40	,,	250
Mincemeat	,,	45	,,	285
PREWETT'S				
Honey & Sesame Spread	1 oz	124	100 g	439
Peanut Butter				
Crunchy & Smooth	,,	169	,,	596
Mincemeat	,,	117	,,	287

Jam, Marmalade, Honey, Spreads

Food	Quantities	Calories	Quantities	Calories
ROBERTSON'S				
Jam – all flavours	1 oz	17	100 g	251
Lemon Curd	"	83	"	291
Marmalade – all varieties	"	71	"	251
Mincemeat, standard	"	75	"	266
Mincemeat, traditional	"	75	"	266
Pure Fruit Spread, all flavours	"	34	"	120
'Today's Recipe'				
Jam, all flavours	"	43	"	150
Marmalade	"	43	"	150
Mincemeat	"	80	"	281
ROSE'S				
Marmalades	1 oz	40	100 g	255
SAFEWAY				
Hazelnut Spread	1 oz	166	100 g	586
Honey – average	"	83	"	291
Jams – average all flavours	"	71	"	253
'No Added Sugar' jams – average	"	40	"	140
Lemon Curd	"	82	"	290
Luxury Mincemeat	"	76	"	269
Marmalade – average	"	71	"	252
Mincemeat	"	76	"	268
Peanut Butter – Smooth/Crunchy	"	170	"	600

Jam, Marmalade, Honey, Spreads

Food	Quantities	Calories	Quantities	Calories
Savoury Spread	1 oz	64	100 g	224
SPAR				
Black Cherry Conserve	1 oz	70	100 g	247
Strawberry Conserve	,,	70	,,	247
SUN-PAT				
Hazelnut Chocolate Spread	1 oz	149	100 g	526
Peanut Butter				
Smooth/Crunch	,,	174	,,	613
Wholenut	,,	175	,,	618
WAITROSE				
Hazelnut Spread	1 oz	150	100 g	530
Fruit Spread – all flavours	,,	35	,,	124
Honey & all flavours	,,	86	,,	304
Jam – average all flavours	,,	70	,,	248
Jam – reduced Sugar	,,	35	,,	124
Lemon Cheese	,,	93	,,	329
Lemon Curd	,,	78	,,	276
Marmalade – all flavours	,,	70	,,	248
Mincemeat	,,	78	,,	275
Peanut Butter	,,	170	,,	600
Stem Ginger in Syrup	,,	74	,,	260

Pasta, Pizza, Rice & Whole Grain Products

Most of the products in this section are useful and healthy on a slimming diet. As long as you check the calorie content carefully and avoid those dishes made with a lot of fat then pasta, rice, whole grains and even pizza are not as fattening as many meat dishes. Pasta has suddenly become fashionable in this country, with fast-food pasta restaurants springing up all over the place. It is now frequently also made with wholewheat flour, which is of course healthier (and tastier). Wholewheat pizza is even available. So ring the changes in your diet by eating more things from this section.

Food	Quantities	Calories	Quantities	Calories
BEJAM *(frozen)*				
Lasagne	1 serving	527		
Pizza				
5″ Cheese & Tomato	1 pizza	234		
5″ Ham & Mushroom	″	225		
Spaghetti Bolognese	1 serving	256		
Vegetable Lasagne	″	374		

Pasta, Pizza, Rice & Whole Grain Products

Food	Quantities	Calories	Quantities	Calories
BE-WELL *(dry)*				
Cereal Savour	1 oz	98	100 g	347
Grain Pilaf	”	97	”	342
Mixed Grain Kasha	”	103	”	364
Mixed Grain Veg. Paella	”	97	”	342
Savoury Couscous	”	97	”	342
Sultan's Pilaf	”	100	”	354
Spicy Whole Grain Couscous	”	92	”	324
Whole Lentil & Barley Pilaf	”	93	”	328
BIRD'S EYE *(frozen)*				
'Menumaster'				
French Bread Pizza	one	330		
Lasagne	9 oz	315		
Pizza				
Tomato & Cheese	93 g	270		
Tomato & Cheese	227 g	630		
Ham & Mushroom	265 g	640		
BUITONI *(tinned)*				
Cannelloni	1 oz	27	100 g	97
Ravioli	”	23	”	82
Wholewheat Ravioli	”	24	”	84
CROSSE & BLACKWELL				
Alphabetti Spaghetti	1 oz	17	100 g	61
Light Spaghetti	”	16	”	57

Pasta, Pizza, Rice & Whole Grain Products

Food	Quantities	Calories	Quantities	Calories
Spaghetti Rings	1 oz	17	100 g	61
Wholewheat Spaghetti	"	18	"	65
Wholewheat Spaghetti Rings	"	16	"	58
Wholewheat Spaghetti Spirals	"	18	"	62
'Pasta Choice'				
Cheese	"	98	"	344
Mushroom	"	99	"	349
Tomato	"	100	"	353
Savoury Curried Rice				
(reconstituted)	"	30	"	105
Savoury Rice & Mushrooms	"	30	"	106
Savoury Rice & Peppers	"	30	"	106
Savoury Rice & Vegetables	"	30	"	105
FINDUS (frozen)				
Cannelloni	1 oz	.34	100 g	119
Lasagne	"	34	"	121
'Crispy Base Pizza'				
Cheese & Tomato	"	59	"	208
Ham	"	48	"	168
'Crusty Bun Pizza'	"	66	"	231
'French Bread Pizza'				
Bacon, Peppers &				
Mushroom	"	54	"	192
Italian Style Sausage	"	52	"	183
Savoury Barbecue	"	63	"	223
Tomato & Cheese	"	65	"	228

Pasta, Pizza, Rice & Whole Grain Products

Food	Quantities	Calories	Quantities	Calories
HEINZ				
Haunted House	1 oz	20	100 g	72
Invaders	"	18	"	65
Invaders with Meateors	"	25	"	89
Ravioli in Beef & Tomato Sauce	"	21	"	76
Ravioli in Tomato Sauce	"	21	"	76
Spaghetti Bolognese	"	23	"	82
Spaghetti Hoops in Tomato Sauce	"	18	"	64
Spaghetti in Tomato Sauce	"	19	"	68
Wholewheat Pasta Shells in Spicy Tomato Sauce	"	18	"	65
JORDANS				
Country Rice & Grains *(dry)*	1 oz	93	100 g	330
KELLOGGS				
Boil in the Bag Rice	1 oz	95	100 g	333
MARKS & SPENCER				
Canneloni	1 oz	38	100 g	133
Cheese/Tomato American-style Pizza	"	60	"	212
Tomato, Cheese & Onion Pizzas frozen	"	58	"	203
Lasagne frozen	"	39	"	136

Pasta, Pizza, Rice & Whole Grain Products

Food	Quantities	Calories	Quantities	Calories
fresh	1 oz	41	100 g	144
Spaghetti Bolognaise (frozen)	"	34	"	121
Tagliatelle – New Style	"	40	"	142

POT CASSEROLE
| Beef | each | 195 | | |

POT NOODLE
Beef and Tomato	each	288		
Cheese & Tomato	"	265		
Chicken & Mushroom	"	289		
Spicy Curry	"	308		
Sweet & Sour	"	269		

POT RICE
Chicken Curry	each	215		
Chicken Risotto	"	195		
Savoury Beef	"	212		

ROSS *(frozen)*
Pasta
| Lasagne | 1 oz | 34 | 100 g | 120 |
| Macaroni Cheese | " | 31 | " | 110 |

Pizza – 4½"
Cheese & Onion	each	190	100 g	210
Crispy Bacon	"	230	"	250
Ham Mushroom & Cheese	"	200	"	220

Pasta, Pizza, Rice & Whole Grain Products

Food	Quantities	Calories	Quantities	Calories
Tomato & Cheese	each	200	100 g	220
Wholemeal, Tomato & Cheese	,,	210	,,	237
French Bread Pizza	,,	380	,,	270
Frozen Rice				
Chinese Special	1 oz	34	100 g	120
Stir Fry Mix	,,	20	,,	70
SAFEWAY				
Tinned				
Macaroni Cheese	1 oz	33	100 g	118
Spaghetti in Tomato Sauce	,,	17	,,	59
Spaghetti Rings in Tomato Sauce	,,	17	,,	59
Dry				
'Savoury Rice				
Chicken & Sweetcorn	,,	100	,,	353
Curry	,,	97	,,	342
Golden Vegetable	,,	95	,,	336
Mixed Vegetables	,,	95	,,	333
Mushroom & Peppers	,,	97	,,	342
Spanish	,,	95	,,	334
Tomato	,,	94	,,	330
Frozen Pizzas				
Cheese & Tomato	,,	70	,,	247
Cheese & Onion	,,	66	,,	233
Ham & Mushroom	,,	64	,,	227

Pasta, Pizza, Rice & Whole Grain Products

Food	Quantities	Calories	Quantities	Calories
Luxury Pizza, Pepperoni	1 oz	58	100 g	205
Luxury Pizza, Tuna and Prawn	"	56	"	198
Pizza 4's	"	65	"	230
Fresh Pizzas				
Cheese, Tomato, Pepper, Onion etc	"	58	"	206
Cheese & Tomato/Onion/ Mushroom	"	61	"	215
Cheese & Tom/Pepper/Ham/ Mushroom	"	58	"	206
Cheese & Tom/Pepperoni & Peppers	"	56	"	198
Swiss Cheese & Ham Deep Dish	"	70	"	246
Tomato, Cheese, Ham Deep Dish	"	56	"	198
Tomato, Cheese, Pineapple & Ham	"	56	"	198
Wholemeal Pizza Bread	"	73	"	258
SAINSBURY				
Frozen pizzas				
Cheese & Tomato Pizza Snacks	each	175	100 g	225
Deep filled Bacon Pizza	1 oz	57	"	200
Deep Filled Chilli Pizza	"	55	"	195

Pasta, Pizza, Rice & Whole Grain Products

Food	Quantities	Calories	Quantities	Calories
Deep Filled Vegetable Pizza	1 oz	57	100 g	200
Italian Style Pizza	½ pizza	420		
Pan Baked Cheese & Tomato	1 oz	58	"	205
Party Pizza Wedges	1 wedge	175	"	225
Ready to eat Meals				
Chilled				
Lasagne Pescatore	1 pack	450		
Lasagne Vegetali	½ pack	160		
Lasagne Verdi	1 serving	375		
Frozen				
Cannelloni	½ pack	250		
Ravioli	1 pack	355		
Spaghetti & Bolognese Sauce	1 oz	37	100 g	130
Tagliatelle	"	37	"	130
Vegetable Lasagne	1 pack	665	"	195
Rice, dry				
'Savoury Rice'				
Brown with Chicken/				
Sweetcorn	1 oz	47	100 g	165
Brown with Fruit/Spice	"	30	"	105
Brown with Peppers/				
Mushrooms	"	38	"	135
Curry	"	47	"	165
Golden Vegetable	"	44	"	155
Saffron	"	45	"	160
Sweet & Sour	"	44	"	155
Tomato Rice	"	44	"	155

Pasta, Pizza, Rice & Whole Grain Products

Food	Quantities	Calories	Quantities	Calories
Tinned				
Ravioli	1 oz	23	100 g	81
Spaghetti	"	16	"	56
WAITROSE				
Pasta Prepared Meals				
Fish Lasagne	1 oz	33	100 g	116
Lasagne	"	41	"	145
Tagliatelle Nicoise	"	48	"	170
Vegetable Lasagne	"	30	"	106
Pizzas				
Chilli Con Carne Pan Bake	"	63	"	222
Campagnola	"	46	"	164
Cheese & Tomato Pan Bake	"	63	"	222
French Bread				
Ham & Mushroom	"	57	"	201
Tomato & Cheese	"	62	"	220
Marinara	"	51	"	179
Pepperoni	"	54	"	189
Tinned				
Ravioli in Meat &				
Tomato Sauce	"	23	"	83
Spaghetti in Tomato Sauce	"	16	"	55
Spaghetti Rings in				
Tomato Sauce	"	17	"	61

Meats, Poultry, Savoury Pies, Sausages, Quiches & Ready-Prepared Main Meals

This is such a huge and diverse section that it cannot be complete. There is such a wide range on the market, which changes almost daily, that you will unfortunately not find every product to be found in your local supermarket in this book. However there is a good selection for you to choose from and do check calories carefully. Some of the dishes do not contain meat but only those which are definitely 'vegetarian' appear in the new section at the very end of the book.

Food	Quantities	Calories	Quantities	Calories
ALLINSON *(dry)*				
Hot Brunch Pot Snack	1 serving	250	100 g	345
Brunch Pot Snack	"	327	"	345
BAXTER *(tinned)*				
Scottish Haggis	1 oz	48	100 g	169

Meats, Poultry, Savoury Pies, Sausages, Quiches

Food	Quantities	Calories	Quantities	Calories
Scotch Mince	1 oz	28	100 g	99
Whole Roast Grouse (boned)	"	49	"	173
Whole Roast Partridge (boned)	"	60	"	212
Whole Roast Pheasant (boned)	"	60	"	213

BEJAM *(frozen)*
Chinese Style

Food	Quantities	Calories	Quantities	Calories
Beef Chop Suey	1 serving	105		
Chicken & Mushroom	"	143		
Chinese Stir-Fry Meal	"	280		
Indian Stir-Fry Meal	"	331		
Oriental Prawn Stir-Fry	"	350		
Ovenable Spring Rolls	each	162		
Prawn Curry	1 serving	85		
Special Fried Rice	"	217		
Sweet 'n' Sour Chicken	"	145		
Sweet 'n' Sour Pork	"	338		

Poultry

Food	Quantities	Calories	Quantities	Calories
Chicken Bites	each	36		
Chicken Cordon Bleu	1 serving	499		
Chicken Kiev	"	648		
Chinese Chicken Wings	1 oz	75	100 g	264
'Goldenbake'				
Cheeseburger	each	251		
Chicken Breast Steak	"	254		

Meats, Poultry, Savoury Pies, Sausages, Quiches

Food	Quantities	Calories	Quantities	Calories
Chicken Drumstick	1 oz	65	100 g	229
Chicken Finger	each	44		
Chicken Nibble	"	120		
Chicken Nugget (no sauce)	"	40		
Chicken Portion	1 oz	59	"	208
Southern-Style Chicken	"	67	"	236
Turkey Steaks	each	164		
Turkey Bites	"	42		
Burgers & Sausages				
100% Beefburgers	each	100		
80% Beefburgers	"	88		
Beefburger with Onion	"	125		
Beefburger, Low Fat	"	95		
Beefburger, Quarterpounder	"	209		
Cocktail	"	34		
Economy Thick Pork	"	148		
Economy Thick Pork & Beef	"	115		
Jumbo Pork & Beef	"	281		
Low-Fat Thick Pork	"	93		
Pork Sausagemeat	"	87		
Premium Pork	"	198		
Thick Beef	"	144		
Thick Pork	"	144		
Thick Pork & Beef	"	150		
Thick Pork & Herbs	"	135		
Thin Pork	"	72		
Thin Pork & Beef	"	75		

Meats, Poultry, Savoury Pies, Sausages, Quiches

Food	Quantities	Calories	Quantities	Calories
Snacks				
Battered Sausages & Chips	1 serving	563		
Chicken & Chips	"	510		
Goldenbake Beef Fingers	each	37		
Goldenbake Lamb Fingers	"	38		
Jumbo Fish Fingers & Chips	"	478		
Pies, Pasties & Sausage Rolls				
Bacon & Cheese Flan	1 flan	316		
Buffet Pork Pies	each	351		
Chicken Bacon &				
Mushroom Flan	1 flan	288		
Chicken & Ham Pies	each	519		
Family Chicken Pie	¼ pie	402		
Family Steak & Kidney Pie	"	459		
Individual Chicken Pie	5 oz pie	385		
Individual Steak & Kidney	"	391		
Mini Cornish Pasty	each	154		
Quiche Lorraine	1 quiche	338		
Sausage Rolls				
Kingsize	each	179		
Party size	"	78		
Savoury Eggs	each	205		
Savoury Minced Beef Roll	½ roll	529		
Traditional Cornish Pasty	each	505		
Turkey & Ham Buffet Pies	"	308		
(Microwave/Ovenbake)				
Beef Curry & Rice	1 serving	472		

Meats, Poultry, Savoury Pies, Sausages, Quiches

Food	Quantities	Calories	Quantities	Calories
Beef Stew & Dumplings	1 serving	446		
Beef Stroganoff & Rice	,,	444		
Cauliflower Cheese	,,	355		
Chicken Chasseur & Rice	,,	362		
Chicken Curry & Rice	,,	432		
Chicken Florentine En-Croute	,,	416		
Chicken Supreme & Rice	,,	456		
Chilli Con Carne	,,	346		
Turkey with Asparagus en Croute	,,	409		
Vegetables au Gratin	,,	285		
BIRD'S EYE				
Beefburgers, 100%	one	120		
Beefburgers, low fat				
grilled	,,	85		
fried	,,	90		
Beefburgers, original	,,	130		
Beef Steak Pie	1 pie	370		
Brunches				
fried	one	155		
grilled	,,	180		
Cheesies				
fried	,,	85		
grilled	,,	75		
Chicklets				
fried	,,	195		

Meats, Poultry, Savoury Pies, Sausages, Quiches

Food	Quantities	Calories	Quantities	Calories
grilled	"	160		
Chicken Pie	serves 1	410		
Chicken Pie	serves 2/3	1075		
Chicken & Mushroom Pie	serves 1	350		
Grills				
Beef	one	185		
Lamb	"	190		
Pancakes				
Cheese & Ham	"	160		
Chicken & Mushroom	"	150		
Minced Beef	"	130		
Prizesteak	"	235		
Quarter Pounders				
fried	"	290		
grilled	"	260		
Sausage Rolls baked	cocktail	65		
Sausage Rolls baked	king	190		
Savoury Rissoles	one	190		
St4eak & Kidney Pie	serves 1	370		
Steak & Kidney Pie	serves 2/3	1120		
Value Grills				
fried	one	190		
grilled	"	175		
Value Grill & Chips				
fried	1 pkt	555		
grilled	"	485		
Value Minced Beef & Veg Pie	serves 1	410		

Meats, Poultry, Savoury Pies, Sausages, Quiches

Food	Quantities	Calories	Quantities	Calories
	serves 2/3	1070		
BIRD'S EYE 'Menumaster'				
Complete Meals				
Gammon Platter	1 pkt	300		
Haddock Platter	"	345		
Prizesteak Platter	"	520		
Roast Beef Platter	"	375		
Roast Chicken Platter	"	360		
Flaky Bake Pies				
Chicken & Ham	one	525		
Seafood	"	445		
Steak & Mushroom	"	505		
International Meals				
Beef Curry with Rice	1 pkt	380		
Beef Oriental	"	310		
Beef Provencale	"	340		
Chicken Curry with Rice	"	400		
Chicken Chow Mein	"	320		
Chicken Risotto	"	455		
Chicken Supreme with Rice	"	460		
Chilli Con Carne with Rice	"	460		
Paella – Seafood & Chicken				
as sold	1 pkt	320		
cooked with butter	"	340		
Prawn Curry with Rice	"	350		
Spaghetti Bolognese	"	370		

Meats, Poultry, Savoury Pies, Sausages, Quiches

Food	Quantities	Calories	Quantities	Calories
Sweet & Sour Pork with Rice	1 pkt	670		
Traditional Meals				
Beef Stew & Dumplings	"	240		
Braised Kidneys in gravy	"	200		
Cheese, Egg & Bacon Flan	5 oz	460		
	11 oz	850		
Cheese, Egg & Onion Flan	5 oz	460		
	11 oz	850		
Chicken & Mushroom Casserole	1 pkt	160		
Faggots in Rich Sauce	10 oz	690		
Lean Roast Beef & Gravy	4 oz pkt	95		
Liver with Onion & Gravy	1 pkt	190		
Macaroni Cheese	"	470		
Minced Beef with Veg in Gravy	1 pkt	150		
Roast Beef Dinner	1 tray	360		
Roast Chicken & Gravy	8 oz pkt	190		
Shepherds Pie	8 oz	270		
Somerset Chicken & Veg. Bake	1 pkt	365		
Vegetable Meals				
Cauliflower Cheese	1 pkt	395		
Mushroom & Pasta Italienne	"	303		
Sweet & Sour Vegetables with Wild Rice	"	285		

Meats, Poultry, Savoury Pies, Sausages, Quiches

Food	Quantities	Calories	Quantities	Calories
Vegetable Chilli with Mexican Rice	1 pkt	340		
Vegetable Curry with Pilau Rice	"	400		
Vegetable Lasagne	"	280		
BRAINS *(frozen)*				
Cottage Pie	½ pie	159	100 g	93
Faggots in Rich Sauce	2	300	"	162
Family Shepherd's Pie	½ pie	214	"	93
CAMPBELL'S *(tinned)*				
Meatballs				
Beef Gravy	1 oz	23	100 g	82
Curry Sauce	"	32	"	114
Onion Gravy	"	24	"	84
Tomato Sauce	"	27	"	96
Quick Snack				
Beef Curry	"	29	"	103
Beef Goulash	"	23	"	80
Chicken Curry	"	24	"	85
Chicken Supreme	"	33	"	116
Chilli Con Carne	"	35	"	124
Stews				
Beef	"	20	"	70
Chicken	"	19	"	66

Meats, Poultry, Savoury Pies, Sausages, Quiches

Food	Quantities	Calories	Quantities	Calories
Minced Beef & Veg.	1 oz	28	100 g	99
Steak & Kidney	”	18	”	64
CROSS & BLACKWELL *(tinned)*				
Baked Beans	1 oz	21	100 g	73
Baked Beans & Hamburgers	”	35	”	122
Baked Beans & Sausages	”	35	”	124
'Cook in the Pot'				
Beef Goulash	”	108	”	380
Beef Stroganoff	”	119	”	418
Chicken Chasseur	”	110	”	389
Chilli-con-Carne	”	108	”	382
Fish Bonne Femme	”	108	”	379
Lamb Ragout	”	110	- ”	389
Madras Curry	”	125	”	442
Ready Meals & Snacks				
Bacon Grill	”	45	”	157
Chicken Curry				
with separate rice	”	31	”	111
Chilli Con Carne	”	35	”	125
Curry with Sep. Rice	”	38	”	135
Macaroni Cheese	”	29	”	102
Faggots 'n' Peas	”	32	”	112
'Cold Meat Products'				
Ham & Beef Roll	”	62	”	220
Ham & Chicken Roll	”	64	”	226
Ham & Tongue roll	”	77	”	270

Meats, Poultry, Savoury Pies, Sausages, Quiches

Food	Quantities	Calories	Quantities	Calories
FINDUS *(frozen)*				
Beefburgers, 100%	1 oz	80	100 g	283
Beef Curry	,,	32	,,	113
Beef Oriental	,,	30	,,	106
Beef Grill Steaks	,,	66	,,	233
Beef Quarter Pounders	,,	80	,,	283
Beef Teriyaki	,,	29	,,	104
Broccoli with Chicken Gratin	,,	42	,,	104
'Crepes'				
Asparagus with Ham	,,	40	,,	141
Beef Burgundy	,,	40	,,	140
Chicken with Mushroom				
Sauce	,,	38	,,	135
Swiss Cheese with Ham	,,	52	,,	182
Chicken Curry	,,	31	,,	110
Cream Chicken with Pasta	,,	41	,,	143
Cumberland Pie	,,	43	,,	153
Egg, Cheese & Bacon Flan	,,	68	,,	239
French Mushroom Flan	,,	64	,,	224
French Onion Flan	,,	66	,,	231
Moussaka	,,	54	,,	190
'Pancakes'				
Cheddar Cheese	,,	54	,,	191
Chicken and Bacon	,,	40	,,	142
Chicken Curry	,,	45	,,	160
Minced Beef	,,	45	,,	159
Smoky Bacon	,,	40	,,	140

Meats, Poultry, Savoury Pies, Sausages, Quiches

Food	Quantities	Calories	Quantities	Calories
'Savoury Toasts'				
Bacon & Egg	1 oz	56	100 g	198
Ham & Cheese	''	62	''	220
Minced Beef	''	56	''	199
Roast Beef in Gravy	''	23	''	82
Shepherds Pie	''	34	''	121
Toad-in-the-Hole	''	59	''	207
Turkey Ragout	''	39	''	138
'Lean Cuisine'				
Bavarian Meatball Casserole	1 oz	23	100 g	81
Beef Julienne	''	28	''	99
Beef & Pork Cannelloni	''	24	''	86
Beef Provencale	''	28	''	100
Chicken à l'Orange	''	34	''	119
Chicken Cacciatore	''	23	''	81
Chicken & Oriental				
Vegetables	''	81		
Glazed Chicken	''	31	''	110
Spaghetti Bolognese	''	21	''	74
Zuccini Lasagne	''	23	''	82
FRAY BENTOS				
(tinned)				
Chicken & Mushroom Pie	1 tin (15 oz)	830	100 g	196
Chicken & Mushroom Pie				
Filling	''	455	''	107
Corned Beef	1 tin (12 oz)	740	''	217

Meats, Poultry, Savoury Pies, Sausages, Quiches

Food	Quantities	Calories	Quantities	Calories
Steak & Ale Pie	1 tin (15 oz)	890	,,	210
Steak & Ale Pudding	,,	955	,,	225
Steak & Kidney Pie Filling	,,	630	,,	148
Steak & Kidney Pie	,,	935	,,	220
Steak & Kidney Pudding	,,	905	,,	212
Steak & Onion Pie Filling	,,	670	,,	158
Steak & Vegetable Pie	,,	775	,,	185
Steak & Vegetable Pie Filling	,,	824	,,	193
Steak & Vegetable Pudding	,,	915	,,	215
Steak with Onion in Ale Gravy	,,	658	,,	155

HARTLEY
| Baked Beans | 1 oz | 18 | 100 g | 65 |

HEINZ
Baked Beans in Barbecue Sauce	1 oz	20	100 g	72
Baked Beans with Pork Sausages	,,	35	,,	124
Baked Beaks in Tomato Sauce	,,	20	,,	72
Curried Beans with Sultanas	,,	15	,,	88

KRAFT *(frozen)*
| Cheese & Onion Pasties | each | 306 | 100 g | 325 |
| Cornish Pasties | ,, | 364 | ,, | 314 |

Meats, Poultry, Savoury Pies, Sausages, Quiches

Food	Quantities	Calories	Quantities	Calories
Country Beef & Vegetable Pies	each	359	100 g	260
Country Chicken Pies	”	389	”	282
Country Chicken & Vegetable Pies	”	386	”	280
Country Steak & Kidney Pies	”	407	”	277
Ploughmans Pasties	”	441	”	304
Sausage Rolls				
Cheese Pastry	”	73	”	332
Cocktail	”	76	”	344
Giant	”	275	”	344
King	”	172	”	344
Party	”	76	”	344
MARKS & SPENCER *(tinned)*				
Beef Stew & Dumplings	1 oz	31	”	110
Beefburgers in Brown Sauce	”	29	”	102
Chicken Curry, mild	”	32	”	112
Chicken in Rich Cream Sauce	”	37	”	132
Chicken with Courgettes/ Honey	”	25	”	90
Chilli Con Carne	”	31	”	110
Chunky Chicken	”	43	”	150
Chunky Curried Beef	”	28	”	99
Chunky Steak in Rich Gravy	”	28	”	100
Curried Chicken, extra strong	”	34	”	120

Meats, Poultry, Savoury Pies, Sausages, Quiches

Food	Quantities	Calories	Quantities	Calories
Irish Stew	1 oz	22	100 g	78
Minced Beef in Rich Gravy	,,	43	,,	150
Moussaka	,,	31	,,	110
Pork Provencal	,,	31	,,	110
Ratatouille	,,	11	,,	39
Steak & Kidney Pudding	,,	45	,,	157
Prepared dishes				
Barbecue Pork Spare Ribs	,,	68	,,	239
Beef Enchiladas	,,	35	,,	123
Beef Stew & Dumplings	,,	42	,,	147
Beef Stroganoff	,,	47	,,	167
Braised Steak	,,	28	,,	100
Chilli con Carne	,,	34	,,	119
Liver & Bacon	,,	39	,,	138
Moussaka	,,	37	,,	132
Pancake-Cheese/Ham, Beer Batter	,,	63	,,	221
Spring Roll – Chinese Style	,,	50	,,	178
Steak & Kidney Pie Meal	,,	57	,,	200
Sweet & Sour Pork Balls	,,	36	,,	128
Burgers, Patés & Sausages				
Beefburgers	,,	74	,,	260
Beefburgers, extra lean	,,	159	,,	560
Beefburgers with onion	,,	74	,,	260
Beef Sausages	,,	106	,,	375
Farmhouse Paté	,,	67	,,	238
Frankfurters	,,	84	,,	295

Meats, Poultry, Savoury Pies, Sausages, Quiches

Food	Quantities	Calories	Quantities	Calories
Pork & Beef Sausages	1 oz	105	100 g	370
Pork & Beef Skinless Sausages	"	71	"	250
Pork Cocktail Sausages	"	99	"	350
Pork Sausages, low fat	"	51	"	180
Pork, Raisin & Orange Stuffing	"	79	"	278
Prize Winning Pork Sausages	"	76	"	268
Saucisson Lyonnaise		N/A		
Schinken Pastete	"	71	"	252
Sliced Scottish Lorne Sausages	"	101	"	355
Top Quality Sausages	"	114	"	400
Minced Beef Pies				
Bolognaise Lattice Pie	"	70	"	245
Minced Beef & Veg Plate Pie	"	75	"	265
Minced Beef Pie (Topcrust)	"	60	"	210
Minced Beef Roll	"	85	"	301
Pasties & pork pies				
Beef & Mushroom Puff Pasty	"	33	"	117
Beef & Onion	"	74	"	262
Cornish Puff Pastry	"	68	"	239
Cornish with Fresh Veg.	"	73	"	258
Lattice Sausage Rolls	"	112	"	396
Melton Mowbray Pork Pie (large)	"	100	"	353
Mini Pastie with Fresh Veg.	"	73	"	258

Meats, Poultry, Savoury Pies, Sausages, Quiches

Food	Quantities	Calories	Quantities	Calories
Pork & Egg Pie	1 oz	92	100 g	324
Pork Pie – cured	,,	99	,,	348
Pork Pie – crisp bake	,,	96	,,	339
Pork Pie & Maltodextrin	,,	99	,,	348
Swiss Pies	,,	84	,,	296
Potato topped pies				
Cottage Pie, Fresh Potato	,,	48	,,	168
– Individual	,,	41	,,	144
Cumberland Pie	,,	48	,,	168
Shepherds Pie – Individual	,,	42	,,	149
Other pies & flans				
Bacon, Egg & Sausage Flan	,,	85	,,	300
Beef/Veg Pie – Suet Pastry	,,	61	,,	215
Chicken & Ham Pie	,,	89	,,	314
Chicken & Ham Pies, mini	,,	89	,,	314
Chicken & Leek Plate Pie	,,	70	,,	248
Chicken & Mushroom Plate Pie	,,	60	,,	212
Chicken Pie, Shortcrust – Individual	,,	82	,,	290
Cocktail Sausage Rolls	,,	114	,,	400
Ground Beef Pie	,,	89	,,	315
Quiche				
Broccoli	,,	66	,,	234
Chicken & Watercress	,,	64	,,	227
Cheese & Tomato	,,	79	,,	280
Cheese & Onion	,,	89	,,	300

Meats, Poultry, Savoury Pies, Sausages, Quiches

Food	Quantities	Calories	Quantities	Calories
Ham, Asparagus, Carrot	1 oz	64	100 g	224
Lorraine	”	81	”	285
Mushroom	”	85	”	300
Roast Chicken Plate Pie	”	72	”	254
Roast Turkey & Ham Plate Pie	”	62	”	220
Scotch Pie	”	80	”	282
Steak & Kidney Pie	”	82	”	290
Steak & Kidney Pie, Rich Pastry	”	87	”	305
Steak & Kidney Pudding – Individual	”	60	”	213
Steak, Onion & Carrot Pudding	”	62	”	220
Turkey Pie, Rich Pastry	”	90	”	318
Vegetable Flan	”	65	”	228
Prepared eggs				
Picnic Eggs	”	83	”	293
Scotch Eggs	”	89	”	315
Poultry				
Breaded Chicken Thighs & Drumsticks	”	82	”	289
Breaded Turkey Burger & Cheese	”	74	”	261
Chicken Bites	”	75	”	264
Chicken Breast Fillets in Breadcrumbs	”	82	”	289

Meats, Poultry, Savoury Pies, Sausages, Quiches

Food	Quantities	Calories	Quantities	Calories
Chicken Goujons	1 oz	68	100 g	239
Chicken Liver Paté	,,	64	,,	224
Chicken Medallions	,,	30	,,	105
Chilli Chicken – Cooked	,,	56	,,	199
Chinese-Style Chicken	,,	65	,,	229
Honey & Mustard Breast Fillets	,,	30	,,	105
Turkey Breast – Pork/ Chestnut	,,	92	,,	323
Turkey Breast Steaks – breaded	,,	58	,,	203
Turkey Roast	,,	21	,,	148
Prepared dishes				
Chicken & Pasta Bake	,,	42	,,	147
Chicken Breast – stuffed/ boneless	,,	57	,,	200
Chicken Casserole	,,	30	,,	105
Chicken Chow Mein	,,	23	,,	82
Chicken Curry	,,	45	,,	159
Chicken Curry with Pilau Rice	,,	27	,,	96
Chicken Fricassee	,,	27	,,	97
Chicken Italienne	,,	49	,,	174
Chicken Kiev	,,	75	,,	263
Chicken Roast	,,	35	,,	124
Chicken Supreme	,,	36	,,	127
Coq Au Vin	,,	40	,,	140

Meats, Poultry, Savoury Pies, Sausages, Quiches

Food	Quantities	Calories	Quantities	Calories
Duckling a l'Orange	1 oz	53	100 g	187
Roast Chicken Leg Meal	,,	34	,,	120
Sweet & Sour Chicken	,,	28	,,	99
Turkey Paupiettes	,,	21	,,	74
Turkey Steak in Mushroom Sauce	,,	32	,,	133
Turkey Steak in White Wine Sauce	,,	42	,,	147

MATTESON *(cold)*

Food	Quantities	Calories	Quantities	Calories
Ardennes Paté	1 oz	110	100 g	389
Black Pudding	,,	100	,,	354
Bratwurst Sausage	,,	95	,,	336
Brussels Paté	,,	115	,,	407
Chicken Liver Paté	,,	72	,,	257
Chicken Roll	,,	95	,,	336
Chopped Pork & Ham	,,	95	,,	336
Frankfurters	,,	100	,,	354
Garlic/German sausage	,,	70	,,	248
Ham Cured Shoulder	,,	34	,,	119
Ham Sausage	,,	40	,,	142
Ham & Tongue Paté	,,	60	,,	212
Honeyglaze Ham	,,	55	,,	195
Liver & Bacon Paté	,,	85	,,	301
Liver & Ham Paté	,,	85	,,	301
Liver Light	,,	49	,,	175
Liver Paté	,,	90	,,	319

Meats, Poultry, Savoury Pies, Sausages, Quiches

Food	Quantities	Calories	Quantities	Calories
Liver Sausage	1 oz	75	100 g	265
Lunch Tongue	"	75	"	265
Maryland Ham	"	30	"	106
Old Smokey	"	30	"	106
Paté Lite				
Ardennes	"	65	"	231
Brussels	"	65	"	231
Pepperami	each	130		
Polony	1 oz	70	100 g	248
Pork Luncheon Meat	"	90	"	319
Pork & Pepper Loaf	"	70	"	248
Scotch Eggs	each	290		
Silverside	1 oz	50	100 g	177
Turkey & Ham Loaf	"	55	"	195
Turkey Paté	"	95	"	336
ROSS *(frozen)*				
Bangers & Mash	1 oz	37	100 g	130
Beef Carbonnade	"	28	"	100
Beef Casserole	"	25	"	90
Beef Curry	"	28	"	100
Beef Wholemeal	"	31	"	110
Breast of Chicken Roll	"	43	"	150
Breast of Turkey Roll	"	28	"	100
Chicken				
à la King	"	28	"	100
Breaded Supreme	"	43	"	150

Meats, Poultry, Savoury Pies, Sausages, Quiches

Food	Quantities	Calories	Quantities	Calories
Casserole	1 oz	20	100 g	70
Curry	"	28	"	100
Fried Drumsticks	"	60	"	210
Oven Bake	"	61	"	215
Provencale	"	20	"	70
Spanish Style	"	20	"	70
with Stuffing & Sausages in Gravy	"	31	"	110
Wholemeal	"	13	"	35
Chilli Con Carne	"	34	"	120
Chinese Chicken	"	23	"	80
Chinese Chicken & Prawn Foo Yung	"	25	"	90
Cottage Pie	"	28	"	100
Faggots with Onions in Rich Sauce	"	45	"	160
Gravy with Sliced Beef	"	25	"	90
Gravy with Sliced Lamb	"	37	"	130
Gravy with Sliced Pork	"	31	"	110
Indian Chicken	"	25	"	90
Italian Beef Bolognaise	"	24	"	85
Lamb Casserole	"	28	"	100
Lamb Stew with Dumplings	"	43	"	150
Lancashire Hot Pot	"	34	"	120
Moussaka	"	25	"	90
Pork & Mushroom Crumble	"	48	"	170
Shepherds Pie	"	31	"	110

Meats, Poultry, Savoury Pies, Sausages, Quiches

Food	Quantities	Calories	Quantities	Calories
Sweet & Sour Pork	1 oz	28	100 g	100
Tandoori Chicken	,,	62	,,	220
Vegetable Curry	,,	23	,,	80
Pies, Quiches & Sausage Rolls				
Beef & Kidney Pie	,,	79	,,	280
Cheese & Onion Quiche	,,	71	,,	250
– Individual	each	465	,,	260
Chicken & Mushroom Pie	1 oz	74	,,	260
Chicken Pasties	each	240	,,	270
Chinese Spring Rolls	,,	140	,,	140
Cocktail Sausage Rolls	,,	75	,,	340
Cornish Pasties	,,	240	,,	270
Family Pies				
Chicken	,,	1285	,,	270
Minced Beef & Onion	,,	1380	,,	290
Steak & Kidney	,,	1285	,,	270
Fisherman's Quiche	1 oz	60	,,	210
Individual Pies				
Beef & Kidney Stewpot	each	490	,,	251
Chicken & Vegetable	,,	410	,,	275
Chicken & Veg. Stewpot	,,	440	,,	224
Steak & Kidney	,,	450	,,	300
Steak & Kidney Pudding	,,	305	,,	215
King Size Sausage Rolls	,,	174	,,	340
Minced Beef & Onion Pie	1 oz	77	,,	270
Quiches				
County Vegetable	,,	54	,,	192

Meats, Poultry, Savoury Pies, Sausages, Quiches

Food	Quantities	Calories	Quantities	Calories
Espagne	1 oz	70	100 g	246
Lorraine	"	65	"	230
Sausage & Egg Pie	"	82	"	290
Sausage Rolls	each	150	"	350
Sausage Rolls, Jumbo	"	255	"	350
Spanish Quiche	1 oz	68	"	240
Steak & Kidney Pie	"	60	"	210
Turkey & Ham Pie	"	74	"	260
Burgers, Ribs & Fries				
American Beefburgers	1 oz	91	100 g	320
Barbecue Ribs	each	255	"	245
Beefburgers Best	"	155	"	260
Beefburgers, Economy	"	140	"	270
Beefburgers 100%	1 oz	94	"	330
Beefburgers, Prime	each	130	"	252
Beefwich	"	115	"	270
Breaded Veal Cutlets	"	320	"	270
Bun Burgers	"	228	"	290
Catergrills	"	115	"	220
Chinese Ribs	"	260	"	220
Fries – Cheese & Onion	"	130	"	140
Grillsteaks	"	285	"	320
Jumbo Grills	"	260	"	220
Jumbo Quarterpounders	"	315	"	265
Kebabs				
Lamb	"	255	"	170
Pork	"	160	"	105

Meats, Poultry, Savoury Pies, Sausages, Quiches

Food	Quantities	Calories	Quantities	Calories
Quick Grills	each	285	100 g	320
Sausages				
Pork 8's	,,	200	,,	340
Pork & Beef 8's	,,	170	,,	285
Pork & Beef Jumbo 8's	,,	340	,,	285
Scotch Fritters				
with Beans	,,	250	,,	240
with Cheese	,,	250	,,	240
with Minced Beef	,,	154	,,	170
SAFEWAY				
Alutikian	1 oz	68	100 g	241
Chicken Spring Roll	,,	51	,,	180
Meat Samosa	,,	80	,,	283
Onion Bhajia	,,	53	,,	187
Vegetable Samosa	,,	68	,,	240
Vegetable Spring Roll	,,	51	,,	178
Burgers, Sausages & Loaves				
Beefburgers	,,	80	,,	282
Beefburgers, Quick Cook	,,	79	,,	278
Beefburgers, Ranch Style	,,	73	,,	256
Beef Loaf	,,	80	,,	283
Breaded Beef Grills	,,	85	,,	300
Breaded Pork Grills	,,	89	,,	314
Burgers, Ranch Style Pork	,,	73	,,	256
Chilli Loaf	,,	53	,,	185
Country Style Pork Sausages	,,	108	,,	380

Meats, Poultry, Savoury Pies, Sausages, Quiches

Food	Quantities	Calories	Quantities	Calories
Cumberland Sausages	1 oz	95	100 g	333
Grillsteaks	"	86	"	301
Hot & Spicy Sausages	"	107	"	375
Pork & Beef Sausages	"	92	"	323
Pork Sausages	"	102	"	358
Pork Loaf	"	80	"	283
Pork & Fried Onion Sausages	"	106	"	374
Pork & Herb Sausages	"	101	"	357
Premium Beef Sausages	"	96	"	339
Premium Pork Sausages	"	108	"	380
Premium Pork Sausage Meat	"	111	"	391
Premium Pork Sausages 90% meat	"	97	"	343
Pies, Pasties & Sausage Rolls				
Beef & Onion Pasty	"	80	"	281
Beef Steak Pie	"	82	"	288
Chicken & Mushroom Pie	"	77	"	272
Cornish Pasty	"	74	"	262
Cottage Pie	"	37	"	130
Hot Pot Pie	"	77	"	272
Meat & Potato Pie	"	76	"	268
Melton Pork Pie	"	109	"	384
Minced Beef & Onion Pie	"	83	"	291
Pork Pie, Individual	"	108	"	381
Potato Cheese & Onion Pasty	"	83	"	291
Sausage Rolls large	"	215	"	757

Meats, Poultry, Savoury Pies, Sausages, Quiches

Food	Quantities	Calories	Quantities	Calories
mini	1 oz	196	100 g	691
Steak & Kidney Pie	454 g	83	”	291
	340 g	76	”	267
	198 g	88	”	309

SAINSBURY
Pies, pasties & flans

Food	Quantities	Calories	Quantities	Calories
Bacon Cheese & Egg Pie	1 oz	90	100 g	317
Baked Mince Beef Roll	½ roll	530	”	300
Beef & Horseradish Pie	1 pie	200	”	320
Chicken Pies (4)	”	410		
Chicken & Ham Pie	1 oz	90	”	317
Chicken & Mushroom Pie	each	405	”	285
Chicken Plate Pie	1 oz	78	”	275
Cornish Pasty, individual		365		
large		630		
Deep filled Chicken & Ham Pie	¼ pie	335		
Deep filled Steak Pie	”	310		
Deep filled Steak & Kidney Pie	”	335		
Fishermans Pie	1 serving	375	”	125
Flans				
Cauliflower Cheese	½ flan	455	”	240
Cheese & Onion	”	460	”	275
Egg Bacon & Mushroom	”	495	”	250
Egg Cheese & Bacon	”	495	”	250

Meats, Poultry, Savoury Pies, Sausages, Quiches

Food	Quantities	Calories	Quantities	Calories
Ham Quiche	½ flan	480	100 g	280
Minced Beef & Tomato	”	560	”	270
Mushroom Quiche	”	460	”	250
Fresh Vegetable Pasty	each	340		
Latticed Beef & Gammon Pie	½ pie	505	”	380
Latticed Pork Cheese & Pickle	”	535	”	410
Melton Mowbray Pie	5 oz	540		
Minced Beef Pie	1 oz	83	”	292
Minced Beef Pies (4)	each	475		
Minced Beef & Onion Pie	¼ pie	400		
Mini Pork Pie	each	220		
Pork Pie	4½ oz	470		
Pork Pie, Buffet	each	275		
Potato Cheese & Onion Pasty	each	390		
Premium Steak Pie	1 oz	77	”	270
Premium Steak & Mushroom Pie	”	78	”	275
Savoury Cornish Pasty	each	360		
Savoury Pie	1/3 pie	350	”	250
Savoury Sausage Roll	each	185		
Sausage Roll, Mini	”	100		
Sausage Roll, Large	”	235		
Shepherds Pie	1 oz	49	”	172
Steak & Kidney Pie	”	67	”	235
Steak & Kidney Pudding	6 oz	435		
Steak & Mushroom Pie	each	365		

Meats, Poultry, Savoury Pies, Sausages, Quiches

Food	Quantities	Calories	Quantities	Calories
Steak Pie	5½ oz	445		
Top Crust Poachers Pie	½ pie	315		
Top Crust Steak & Kidney Pie	½ pie	350		
Top Crust Steak & Mushroom Pie	"	430		
Vegetable Pie	1 serving	300		
Burgers, fries, grills				
Beefburgers	each	130		
Beefburgers, low fat	"	75		
Chicken Nuggets & Chips	1 serving	465		
Grillsteaks	each	325		
Sausages				
Beef	each	160		
Cumberland Pork	"	180		
Large Pork & Beef	"	125		
Low Fat Pork	"	100		
Party Pork & Beef	"	45		
Party Pork & Bacon	"	45		
Pork	"	210		
Pork Sausage Meat	1 oz	100	100 g	351
Pork & Beef	each	180		
Premium Pork with Herbs	"	65		
Premium Pork Sausagemeat	1 oz	84	"	295
Skinless Pork	each	100		
Skinless Pork & Beef	"	75	"	305
Frozen sausages				

Meats, Poultry, Savoury Pies, Sausages, Quiches

Food	Quantities	Calories	Quantities	Calories
Economy Pork Sausagemeat	1 oz	87	,,	305
Low Fat Sausages	each	100	,,	235
Lincolnshire Pork	,,	145	,,	340
Thick	,,	155	,,	310
Thin	,,	45	,,	315
Pork Economy, Thick	,,	160	,,	290
Thin	,,	85	,,	340
Pork & Beef, Thick	,,	165	,,	295
Thin	,,	80	,,	295
Premium Pork/Herb	,,	155	,,	275
Premium Pork, Thick	,,	155	,,	280
Delicatessen Department				
Bacon and Ham Loaf	1 oz	60	,,	211
Black Pudding	,,	65	,,	229
Brawn	,,	55	,,	194
Chopped Ham Roll	,,	50	,,	176
Frankfurter				
small	each	70		
large	,,	210		
Ham	1 oz	45	,,	158
Krajana, Polish	,,	35	,,	123
Liver Sausage	,,	80	,,	282
Paté				
low fat Bacon & Liver	1 oz	43	100 g	153
low fat Duck & Orange	,,	61	,,	215
low fat Farmhouse	,,	55	,,	195
low fat Ham	,,	41	,,	144

Meats, Poultry, Savoury Pies, Sausages, Quiches

Food	Quantities	Calories	Quantities	Calories
low fat Liver	1 oz	44	100 g	156
Normandy	"	91	"	320
Paté de Foie	"	88	"	310
Smoked Salmon	"	47	"	165
Mortadella	"	100	"	251
Pork Luncheon Meat	"	80	"	282
Pork Breakfast Sausage	"	70	"	246
Salami, Danish	"	155	"	546
Smoked Pork Sausage with garlic	"	64	"	225
Ready prepared meals				
Chilled				
Barbecue Beef & Egg Fried Rice	1 pack	575	"	125
Barbecue Spare Ribs	1 oz	40	"	140
Beef & Veg Stew with Dumplings	1 pack	530	"	155
Chicken & Ratatouille Bake	"	305	"	90
Chicken Leek & Broccoli Bake	"	480	"	140
Chicken Madras	1 serving	780	"	165
Chilli con Carne	"	227	"	103
Moussaka	"	475	"	85
Traditional Beef Hot Pot	½ pack	340	"	120
Frozen				
Beef Curry & Rice	1 pack	510	"	130
Chicken Curry & Rice	"	410	"	105

Meats, Poultry, Savoury Pies, Sausages, Quiches

Food	Quantities	Calories	Quantities	Calories
Chicken Kiev	1 kiev	610	100 g	305
Chicken Supreme & Rice	1 serving	360	"	95
Chilli con Carne & Rice	"	360	"	95
Moussaka	1 oz	22	"	80
Party Size Vegetable Rolls	each	35	"	310
Stir Fry Chicken & Oriental Vegetables	1 oz	34	"	120
Stir Fry Seafood/Chicken Paella	"	37	"	130
Tinned				
Beef Curry	1 oz	30	"	105
Chicken Curry	"	35	"	125
Chicken in White Sauce	7 oz	325		
Chilli con Carne	1 oz	30	"	105
Chopped Ham & Pork	"	65	"	230
Corned Beef	"	60	"	210
Ham	"	35		
Hot Dogs	each	50	"	215
Irish Stew	15 oz	375		
Minced Beef & Onion	"	300		
Stewed Steak & Gravy	"	735		
SPAR				
Tinned				
Chilli con Carne	1 oz	29	100 g	104
Hot Dog Sausages	"	56	"	197
Irish Stew	"	34	"	119

Meats, Poultry, Savoury Pies, Sausages, Quiches

Food	Quantities	Calories	Quantities	Calories
Minced Beef	1 oz	38	100 g	135
Stewed Steak	"	41	"	144
WAITROSE				
Burgers				
Beefburgers (8 oz)	1 oz	70	100 g	246
Burgersteaks, English	"	82	"	290
Quarter Pounders	"	96	"	338
Cold Meats				
Chicken Paté,				
Gelatine Topped	"	58	"	205
Chicken Roll	"	39	"	136
Continental Honey Roast				
Ham	"	45	"	158
Corned Beef	"	61	"	215
Danish Salami	"	148	"	520
Farmhouse Paté,				
Gelatine Topped	"	62	"	220
Garlic Salami, Single	"	100	"	352
Garlic Sausage	"	74	"	262
German Salami	"	121	"	427
Ham	"	29	"	103
Ham, Buckingham	"	38	"	134
Ham, Honey Roast	"	38	"	134
Ham, Smoked	"	38	"	134
Krakowska	"	75	"	264
Pepper Salami	"	44	"	427

Meats, Poultry, Savoury Pies, Sausages, Quiches

Food	Quantities	Calories	Quantities	Calories
Pork Luncheon Meat	1 oz	101	100 g	356
Roast Loin of Pork	,,	44	,,	156
Shoulder	,,	35	,,	124
Smoked Pork Sausage	,,	93	,,	328
Smoked Viennas	,,	82	,,	290
Turkey Breast Roll	,,	41	,,	144
Pies, quiches & sausage rolls				
Beef en Croute	1 oz	50	100 g	207
Bolognaise Pie	,,	62	,,	220
Chicken & Broccoli	,,	42	,,	147
Chicken, Ham & Mushroom	,,	73	,,	258
Chicken & Vegetable	,,	70	,,	'247
Chunky Chicken with Bacon & Ham	,,	86	,,	302
Chunky Steak with Kidney	,,	82	,,	298
Cottage Pie	,,	39	,,	136
Farmhouse Pork	,,	67	,,	237
Gala Pork, Ham & Egg	,,	63	,,	221
Minced Beef Pie (large)	,,	76	,,	269
(individual)	,,	70	,,	246
Minced Beef & Onion Pie				
(large)	,,	80	,,	282
(individual)	,,	76	,,	269
Pork Pie				
Individual	,,	107	,,	377
Melton Mowbray (1 lb)	,,	114	,,	403
Melton Mowbray (10 oz)	,,	126	,,	444

Meats, Poultry, Savoury Pies, Sausages, Quiches

Food	Quantities	Calories	Quantities	Calories
Mini	1 oz	107	100 g	308
Minced Beef Rolls	,,	107	,,	308
with Mustard	,,	95	,,	333
with Cheese, Ham, Herb	,,	83	,,	293
Quiches				
Broccoli & Swiss Cheese	,,	57	,,	200
Ham & Swiss Cheese	,,	57	,,	200
Mini	,,	81	,,	285
Sausage Rolls	,,	122	,,	430
Savoury Minced Beef Pasties	,,	75	,,	264
Steak & Kidney Pie (1 lb)	,,	76	,,	269
Steak & Kidney Pie (individual)	,,	70	,,	247
Steak & Kidney Pudding (individual)	,,	71	,,	250
Steak, Mushroom & Red Wine Pie	,,	68	,,	239
Turkey & Asparagus en Croute	,,	67	,,	235
Ready Prepared Meals				
Aubergine Gratin	,,	52	,,	185
Beef Cobbler	,,	46	,,	161
Beef Meatballs with Provencale Sauce	,,	76	,,	269
Beef Vindaloo	,,	51	,,	181
Braised Steak	,,	31	,,	109
Cauliflower Cheese	,,	21	,,	76

Meats, Poultry, Savoury Pies, Sausages, Quiches

Food	Quantities	Calories	Quantities	Calories
Chicken & Broccoli with Rice	1 oz	27	100 g	95
Chicken à la King	"	31	"	105
Chicken with Almonds	"	51	"	181
Chicken Biryani	"	33	"	115
Chicken Moghlai	"	57	"	201
Chicken Masala	"	44	"	154
Chicken Tikka	"	49	"	173
Chilli Con Carne	"	25	"	88
Irish Stew	"	30	"	105
Lamb Boulangere	"	48	"	171
Lamb Rogan Josh	"	38	"	136
Leek, Bacon & Tomato Savoury	"	22	"	78
Moussaka	"	51	"	180
Pancakes				
Cheese, Ham & Mushroom	"	45	"	160
Potato, Cheese & Asparagus	"	44	"	156
Pilau Rice	"	129	"	453
Potato Dauphinoise	"	41	"	144
Potato, Onion & Ham Bake	"	31	"	108
Potato Shells				
with Cheese, Ham & Mushroom	"	35	"	125
with Courgettes Provencale	"	31	"	110
Sausages & Mash	"	40	"	140

Meats, Poultry, Savoury Pies, Sausages, Quiches

Food	Quantities	Calories	Quantities	Calories
Shepherds Pie	1 oz	35	100 g	125
Somerset Pie	,,	30	,,	106
Spicy Meatballs	,,	43	,,	150
Sweet & Sour Pork	,,	34	,,	121
Vegetable Pulao	,,	38	,,	135
Sausages				
Beef	,,	65	,,	229
Chipolata	,,	93	,,	326
Cotswold Pork	,,	68	,,	240
Cumberland Pork	,,	77	,,	273
Cumberland Pork Chipolatas	,,	91	,,	320
Cumberland Pork Rings	,,	67	,,	235
Pork Sausages	,,	81	,,	287
Pork, Large	,,	45	,,	159
Pork Meat	,,	81	,,	287
Pork Cocktail	,,	81	,,	287
Pork & Beef	,,	95	,,	335
Pork & Beef Chipolatas	,,	95	,,	335
Pork Cocktail	,,	75	,,	265
Pork Meat	,,	77	,,	270
Premium Beef	,,	65	,,	229
Premium Pork Chipolatas	,,	88	,,	310
Premium Pork	,,	88	,,	310
Spiced Pork	,,	83	,,	292
Suffolk	,,	72	,,	254
Thick Pork	,,	77	,,	270
Thin Pork	,,	78	,,	275

Meats, Poultry, Savoury Pies, Sausages, Quiches

Food	Quantities	Calories	Quantities	Calories
Tinned				
Baked Beans	1 oz	26	100 g	91
in Barbeque Sauce	"	26	"	91
in Chili Sauce	"	27	"	95
in Curry Sauce	"	29	"	101
in Tomato Sauce				
(no added sugar)	"	23	"	81
Snacks				
Chicken Sate Sticks	"	44	"	156
Crespolini in a Pottery Bowl	"	37	"	130
Indian Style Chicken Nibbles	"	20	"	70
Pakora	"	64	"	226
Pork Sate Stick	"	45	"	160
Sate Sauce	"	47	"	165
Smokey Barbeque				
Chicken Nibbles	"	20	"	70
WALLS *(chilled)*				
Chicken & Mushroom Pie	each	365		
Cornish Pasty	"	445		
Grosvenor Pork Pie	113 g slice	410		
Melton Mowbray Pork Pie	each	610		
Minced Beef & Onion Pie	"	470		
Party Pork Pie	"	240		
Pork Pie	"	585		
Sausage Roll	"	145		
Scotch Pie	1 oz	68	100 g	241

Meats, Poultry, Savoury Pies, Sausages, Quiches

Food	Quantities	Calories	Quantities	Calories
Steak & Kidney Pie *(frozen)*	each	455		
Bacon Steak				
in Cheese & Onion Sauce	150 g	210		
in Mushroom Sauce	”	210		
in Parsley Sauce	”	220		
in Savoury Tomato Sauce	”	175		
Sausages				
Light & Lean				
Country	1 oz	56	100 g	198
Premium	”	50	”	178
Thick & Chips	”	54	”	190
Lincolnshire Style	each	113		
Pork Thick & Chips	1 oz	104	”	367
Pork & Beef	”	80	”	282
Smithfield Grills	”	59	”	208
YOUNG'S *(frozen)*				
Chicken Cordon Bleu	1 oz	54	100 g	190
Chicken Kiev	”	67	”	235

Salads

It is, naturally, safer and healthier to prepare your own salads because you can then be sure of the freshness of the ingredients and the amount of oil or mayonnaise in the dressing. There is, however, a wide range of the most delicious and tempting prepared salads around today. They do make an excellent 'packed' lunch to take to work as a change from cottage cheese and crispbread!

Food	Quantities	Calories	Quantities	Calories
CHAMBOURCY				
Coleslaw	1 oz	43	100 g	150
EDEN VALE SALADS				
American	1 oz	40	100 g	142
Coleslaw				
Classic	"	36	"	127
Coarse Cut	"	35	"	124
Diet	"	16	"	55

Food	Quantities	Calories	Quantities	Calories
Fruity	1 oz	59	100 g	207
Mild	,,	57	,,	200
Spicy	,,	57	,,	201
Continental	,,	53	,,	186
Harvest	,,	42	,,	148
Pasta	,,	56	,,	197
Potato & Chive	,,	46	,,	163
Potato, Mild	,,	64	,,	224
Prawn	,,	44	,,	155
Spanish	,,	32	,,	112
Vegetable	,,	40	,,	141
Vegetable, Mild	,,	59	,,	208
Vinaigrette, Diet	,,	9	,,	33
HEINZ *(tinned)*				
Coleslaw	,,	36	,,	126
Potato Salad	,,	48	,,	168
Vegetable Salad	,,	43	,,	152
MARKS & SPENCER				
Carrot & Nut Salad	,,	72	,,	253
Cauliflower & Apple Salad	,,	69	,,	244
Chefs Salad Meal – Paysanne	,,	39	,,	136
Coleslaw	,,	49	,,	172
Coleslaw with Cheese & Chives	,,	81	,,	286
Florida Salad	,,	58	,,	205

Salads

Food	Quantities	Calories	Quantities	Calories
Three Bean Salad	1 oz	42	100 g	148
Waldorf Salad	"	85	"	301
ST IVEL				
Coleslaw	1 oz	35	100 g	125
Prawn Salad	"	44	"	155
SAFEWAY				
Apple & Sultana Coleslaw	1 oz	57	100 g	202
Apple, Raisin				
& Walnut Salad	"	32	"	114
Calorie Reduced Coleslaw	"	15	"	223
Chinese Leaf				
& Sweetcorn Salad	"	13	"	47
Coleslaw Salad	"	57	"	200
Fresh Ratatouille Vegetables	"	16	"	56
Low Calorie Coleslaw	"	57	"	200
Mixed Salad with				
Beansprouts	"	16	"	56
Potato Salad	"	57	"	200
Rice & Chicken Salad	"	61	"	216
Shredded Cabbage,				
White and Red	"	18	"	62
Spanish Salad	"	48	"	169
Special Waldorf Salad	"	73	"	258
Spicy Potato Salad	"	57	"	201
Stir Fry Courgettes	"	24	"	86

Food	Quantities	Calories	Quantities	Calories
Stir Fry Mushrooms	1 oz	23	100 g	80
Vegetable Salad	''	59	''	208
SAINSBURY				
Apple Peach & Nut Salad	1 oz	60	100 g	210
Brown Rice Salad	''	62	''	220
Cheese Celery & Pineapple Salad	''	51	''	180
Celery Apple & Mandarin Salad	''	40	''	140
Coleslaw	''	27	''	95
Coleslaw in Mild Curried Dressing	''	34	''	120
Coleslaw in Reduced Calorie Dressing	''	17	''	45
Crisp Vegetable Salad	''	13	''	45
Mild Curried Rice Salad	''	50	''	175
Potato Celery & Dill Salad	''	37	''	130
Potato Ham & Stilton Salad	''	61	''	215
Sweetcorn Salad	''	38	''	135
Three Bean Salad	''	44	''	155
Vegetable Salad Mix & Rice	''	17	''	60
WAITROSE				
Carnival	1 oz	36	100 g	126
Coleslaw	''	36	''	128
Coleslaw, Cottage	''	83	''	300

Salads

Food	Quantities	Calories	Quantities	Calories
Coleslaw, Low Calorie	1 oz	18	100 g	62
Florida	"	46	"	163
Pasta Romana	"	86	"	303
Potato & Frankfurter	"	85	"	300
Potato & Onion	"	40	"	141
Raita	"	26	"	93
Seafood	"	62	"	220
Tabbouleh	"	40	"	141
Waldorf	"	116	"	407

Sauces, Pickles and Salad Dressings

Sauces and pickles do add variety to a slimming diet and, if used in limited quantities, are not very high in calories. It is, however, all too easy to cheat and pour on several ounces so *measure carefully*. Particularly dangerous are salad dressings and mayonnaise which have a very high oil content. You can now buy reduced calorie mayonnaise and even oil free salad dressing. Inevitably the latter is not nearly as good as the fattening sort but it is useful. (These products are not listed in this book for the usual reason, that their contents appear on their packaging.)

Food	Quantities	Calories	Quantities	Calories
BAXTER'S				
Pickles				
Beetroot in Redcurrant Jelly	1 oz	46	100 g	162
Beetroot				
Baby/Rosebud	”	11	”	39

Sauces, Pickles and Salad Dressings

Food	Quantities	Calories	Quantities	Calories
Crinkle/Sliced	1 oz	9	100 g	34
Shredded	"	10	"	36
Jellied Cranberry Sauce	"	40	"	142
Mint Jelly	"	71	"	252
Mint Sauce	"	33	"	118
Mixed Fruit Chutney	"	43	"	152
Tomato Chutney	"	45	"	161
Whole Fruit Cranberry Sauce	"	39	"	140
Tinned Sauces				
Burgundy Wine	"	15	"	55
Medium Curry	"	21	"	73
Provencale	"	33	"	117
Sweet & Sour	"	25	"	90
White Wine	"	28	"	98
BONNE CUISINE				
Au Poivre	1 oz	109	100 g	383
Basquaise	"	102	"	360
Chasseur	"	98	"	345
Hollandaise	"	109	"	384
Madeira	"	102	"	359
Paysan	"	99	"	348
BRANSTON				
Fruity Sauce	1 oz	25	100 g	90
Onion Relish	"	38	"	135
Spicy Sauce	"	32	"	112

Food	Quantities	Calories	Quantities	Calories
Sweet Pickles	1 oz	37	100 g	131
Sweetcorn Relish	"	38	"	133
Tomato Relish	"	37	"	131
Tomato & Pepper Relish	"	36	"	126
BUITONI				
Bolognese	1 oz	14	100 g	51
Milanese	"	13	"	47
Napolitan	"	7	"	24
Siciliana	"	21	"	74
BURGESS				
Creamed Horsradish	1 oz	54	100 g	190
High Oil Mayonnaise	"	217	"	765
Hot Horseradish Sauce	"	35	"	125
Mango Chutney	"	63	"	221
Mayonnaise	"	168	"	592
Prawn Cocktail Sauce	"	93	"	326
Salad Cream	"	92	"	323
Sauce Tartare	"	80	"	283
Sweet Pickle	"	61	"	215
CAMPBELL'S				
'Spaghetti Sauces'				
Bolognese	1 oz	25	100 g	90
Siciliana	"	20	"	70
Tomato & Mushroom	"	19	"	68

Sauces, Pickles and Salad Dressings

Food	Quantities	Calories	Quantities	Calories
'Prego Sauces'				
Bolognese	1 oz	28	100 g	98
Cacciatore	"	10	"	37
Pizza Topping	"	21	"	76
Piaziola	"	10	"	37
Romagna	"	18	"	64
Tuscany	"	30	"	106
Vino Bianco	"	12	"	43
COLMAN'S				
'Prepared Mustards'				
American	1 oz	31	100 g	110
Dijon	"	48	"	170
French	"	32	"	115
German	"	38	"	135
Horseradish	"	40	"	140
Mild Burger	"	31	"	110
Whole Grain	"	41	"	145
'Condiments'				
Apple Sauce	"	23	"	80
Cranberry & Wine Sauce	"	61	"	215
Creamed Horseradish	"	56	"	200
Fresh Garden Mint Sauce	"	3	"	10
Horseradish Relish	"	28	"	100
Mint Jelly	"	75	"	265
Prawn Cocktail Sauce	"	107	"	380
Redcurrant Cocktail Sauce	"	82	"	290

Sauces, Pickles and Salad Dressings

Food	Quantities	Calories	Quantities	Calories
Sauce Tartare	1 oz	72	100 g	255
'Cooking Mixes'				
Beef Bourguignon	”	99	”	350
Beef Goulash	”	78	”	275
Beef Stroganoff	”	90	”	320
Chicken Chasseur	”	69	”	245
Chilli con Carne	”	83	”	295
Coq au Vin	”	69	”	245
Farmhouse Lamb	”	92	”	325
Korma Mild Curry	”	95	”	335
Liver Casserole	”	99	”	350
Madras Medium Curry	”	95	”	335
Pork Casserole	”	83	”	295
Sausage Casserole	”	97	”	345
Traditional Beef Casserole	”	90	”	320
Traditional Chicken Casserole	”	95	”	335
'Pour Over'				
Apple	”	107	”	380
Bread	”	90	”	320
Cheddar Cheese	”	117	”	415
Cheese with Chives	”	104	”	370
Mushroom	”	95	”	335
Onion	”	93	”	330
Parsley	”	102	”	360
White	”	107	”	380

Sauces, Pickles and Salad Dressings

Food	Quantities	Calories	Quantities	Calories
'Pour-Over' or 'Cook-In'	1 oz	88	100 g	310
Barbecue	"	88	"	310
Beef Seasoning	"	89	"	315
Chicken Seasoning	"	102	"	360
Curry	"	99	"	350
Quick Chilli	"	95	"	335
Spaghetti Bolognese	"	105	"	370
Sweet & Sour	"	90	"	320
CROSSE & BLACKWELL				
Salad Cream	"	98	"	346
Tomato Ketchup	"	33	"	118
'Toss 'n Serve'				
Classic	"	62	"	219
Herb	"	3	"	11
'Pour Over'				
Bolognaise	"	20	"	70
Curry	"	27	"	95
Cheese	"	30	"	106
Sweet & Sour	"	32	"	112
'Dish of the Day'				
Barbecue	"	108	"	382
Bolognese	"	100	"	353
Chilli	"	105	"	370
Garlic & Herb	"	130	"	457
Mild Mustard	"	112	"	394
Southern Style	"	131	"	461

Sauces, Pickles and Salad Dressings

Food	Quantities	Calories	Quantities	Calories
Tandoori	1 oz	131	100 g	461
Tomato & Herb	,,	107	,,	377
DUCHESSE				
Mayonnaise-Style Dressing	1 teaspoon	60	100 ml	450
Low Cholesterol Dressing	,,	60	,,	420
Sunflower Dressing	,,	60	,,	430
Oil-free Dressing	2 teaspoons	1	,,	8
HAYWARDS 'Pickles				
Beetroot	1 oz	11	100 g	40
Gherkins	,,	1	,,	5
Military Pickle	,,	37	,,	130
Mixed Pickle	,,	2	,,	9
Onion	,,	4	,,	16
Piccalilli	,,	8	,,	29
Pickled Dill Gherkins	,,	1	,,	5
Red Cabbage	,,	3	,,	10
Silverskin Onions	,,	6	,,	25
Sweet Piccalilli	,,	21	,,	75
Sweet Pickled Onions	,,	7	,,	25
Walnuts	,,	23	,,	80
HEINZ				
Apple Sauce	1 oz	18	100 g	65
'All Seasons Dressings'				
Cucumber Dressing	,,	78	,,	276

Sauces, Pickles and Salad Dressings

Food	Quantities	Calories	Quantities	Calories
Herb & Garlic	1 oz	86	100 g	302
Mild Curry	,,	78	,,	276
Spring Onion	,,	75	,,	264
Thousand Island	,,	80	,,	282
Yogurt & Chive	,,	83	,,	291
French Dressing	,,	145	,,	511
Mayonnaise	,,	150	,,	530
Ploughman's Ideal Sauce	,,	30	,,	106
Ploughman's Mild Mustard Pickle	,,	32	,,	114
Ploughman's Piccalilli	,,	24	,,	85
Ploughman's Pickle	,,	34	,,	120
Ploughman's Tangy Pickle Spread	,,	33	,,	118
Ploughman's Tomato Pickle	,,	27	,,	95
Salad Cream	,,	97	,,	342
Silverskin Onions	,,	4	,,	13
Tomato and Onion Spread	,,	62	,,	218
Tomato Ketchup	,,	27	,,	97
HELLMAN'S				
Mayonnaise	1 oz	204	100 g	718
Garlic Mayonnaise	,,	204	,,	718
Lemon Mayonnaise	,,	204	,,	718
Reduced Calorie Mayonnaise	,,	83	,,	292
KNORR 'Mixes'				
Apple	1 pkt	98	100 g	349

Sauces, Pickles and Salad Dressings

Food	Quantities	Calories	Quantities	Calories
Bread	1 pkt	132	100 g	368
Cheese	”	134	”	434
Chilli	”	178	”	382
Garlic	”	157	”	435
Goulash	”	169	”	380
Korma Curry	”	176	”	382
Onion	”	96	”	343
Parsley	”	70	”	348
Red Wine	”	117	”	355
Savoury White	”	72	”	360
Spaghetti	”	154	”	334
White Wine	”	175	”	426
'Pasta Sauces'				
Carbonara	”	175	”	492
Napoli	”	159	”	345
Romana	”	168	”	342
'Stuffing Mixes'				
Apricot & Sultana	”	293	”	326
Cider Apple & Herbs	”	361	”	401
Garlic & Herbs	”	370	”	411
Hazelnut & Herbs	”	385	”	428
Muesli	”	327	”	385
Sage, Onion & Bacon	”	364	”	404
'Marinades'				
American Barbecue	”	151	”	328
Country Chicken/Pork	”	84	”	290
Greek Kebab	”	85	”	275
Spicy Lamb/Beef	”	117	”	279

Sauces, Pickles and Salad Dressings

Food	Quantities	Calories	Quantities	Calories
Tandoori	1 pkt	70	100 g	211
'Stock Powder & Cubes'				
Beef Stock Powder	1 pint	17		
Chicken Stock Powder	"	17		
Beef Cube	1 cube	35		
Chicken Cube	"	36		
Gravy Cube	"	41		
Ham Cube	"	28		
Lamb Cube	"	35		
Vegetable Cube	"	34		
KRAFT				
Blue Cheese Dressing	1 oz	137	100 g	482
Classic French Dressing	"	141	"	496
Coleslaw Dressing	"	127	"	449
Italian Garlic Dressing	"	121	"	426
Miracle Whip Dressing	"	125	"	440
Reduce Calorie Vinaigrette	"	25	"	88
Thousand Island Dressing	"	112	"	393
'LIFE' ALL-NATURAL				
Mayonnaise-Style Dressing	1 oz	142	100 g	508
Salad Cream-Style Dressing	"	77	"	275
Tomato Ketchup	"	21	"	76

LYON'S MAID
'Dessert Sauces'

Sauces, Pickles and Salad Dressings

Food	Quantities	Calories	Quantities	Calories
Butterscotch	1 oz	89	100 g	314
Chocolate	"	80	"	283
Raspberry	"	75	"	266
Strawberry	"	75	"	264
MARKS & SPENCER				
Bolognese	1 oz	21	100 g	73
Cream of Mushroom	"	23	"	81
French Salad Dressing	"	196	"	690
Medium Curry Cooking Sauce	"	12	"	41
Napoletana	"	15	"	53
Red Wine Cooking Sauce	"	16	"	55
Sweet & Sour Cooking Sauce	"	11	"	38
'Chutney & Pickles'				
Mango Chutney	"	60	"	210
Pickled Onions	"	6	"	23
Pickled Sliced Beetroot	"	16	"	55
Pickled Small Whole Beetroot	"	16	"	55
'Salad Dressings'				
Creme Fraiche	"	83	"	292
Curry	"	93	"	327
French	"	146	"	515
Herb	"	30	"	105
Italian Style Garlic	"	39	"	138

Sauces, Pickles and Salad Dressings

Food	Quantities	Calories	Quantities	Calories
Marie Rose	1 oz	210	100 g	740
Mayonnaise, fresh	”	214	”	735
Mayonnaise, Low Calorie	”	85	”	298
Sour Cream – Onion	”	109	”	385
Thousand Isle	”	80	”	281
O.K. SAUCES				
Fruity	1 oz	25	100 g	90
Mint	”	11	”	40
Spicy	”	27	”	95
PAN YAN				
Bramley Apple Sauce	1 oz	34	100 g	121
Cranberry Sauce	”	37	”	132
Curried Fruit Chutney	”	41	”	144
Mango Chutney	”	56	”	196
Olde English Chutney	”	50	”	176
Original Pickle	”	38	”	133
Piccalilli	”	19	”	68
Sweet & Sour Pickle	”	39	”	139
PREWETT'S				
Ketchup	1 oz	12	100 g	44
Mayonnaise Style Dressing	”	137	”	482
Salad Cream Style Dressing	”	78	”	275
Spicy Brown Sauce	”	29	”	102

Sauces, Pickles and Salad Dressings

Food	Quantities	Calories	Quantities	Calories
SAFEWAY				
French Oil Dressing	1 oz	137	100 g	481
Garlic Oil Dressing	”	126	”	443
Italian Oil Dressing	”	126	”	443
Mayonnaise				
American Style	”	214	”	755
Garlic	”	208	”	734
Lemon	”	208	”	732
Mild Curry	”	208	”	732
Mustard	”	209	”	735
Mustard Oil Dressing	”	129	”	453
Reduced Calorie Dressing	”	44	”	155
Salad Cream	”	92	”	324
Seafood Dressing	”	92	”	324
'Chilled Yoghurt Dressings'				
Blue Cheese	”	93	”	328
Herb & Garlic	”	89	”	314
Tartare Sauce	”	63	”	222
1000 Island	”	77	”	273
Sauces				
*Beef Bourgignon Mix	”	81	”	285
Beef Casserole	”	75	”	265
Bolognese	”	17	”	59
* Bread Sauce Mix	”	100	”	352
*Cheese Sauce Mix	”	126	”	445
*Cheese, Onion				
& Chive Sauce	”	123	”	435

Sauces, Pickles and Salad Dressings

Food	Quantities	Calories	Quantities	Calories
*Chicken Casserole Mix	1 oz	75	100 g	265
*Chicken Chasseur Mix	"	82	"	290
Chilli Con Carne	"	79	"	280
Cranberry	"	39	"	137
Creamed Horseradish	"	52	"	185
*Curry Sauce Mix	"	89	"	315
Fruity Sauce	"	28	"	98
Mint Sauce	"	5	"	18
*Mushroom Sauce Mix	"	111	"	390
*Onion Sauce Mix	"	103	"	364
*Parsley Sauce Mix	"	101	"	356
*Sausage Casserole Mix	"	77	"	270
*Spaghetti Bolognese Mix	"	82	"	290
*Sweet & Sour Sauce Mix	"	92	"	325
Spicy Sauce	"	27	"	94
Tartare Sauce	"	89	"	315
Tomato Ketchup	"	36	"	126
*White Sauce Mix	"	104	"	366

NB: All Dry Weight *

Pickles

Baby Beetroot	"	7	"	26
Chunky Sweet Piccalilli	"	28	"	98
Clear Mixed Pickle	"	2	"	8
Continental Pickle	"	5	"	19
Corn Relish	"	33	"	118
Cucumber Relish	"	33	"	118
Mixed Pickles	"	5	"	19

Sauces, Pickles and Salad Dressings

Food	Quantities	Calories	Quantities	Calories
Mustard Piccalilli	1 oz	10	100 g	35
Mustard Relish	"	33	"	118
Pickled Gherkins	"	2	"	6
Pickled Onions	"	10	"	37
Pickled Sliced Cucumbers	"	8	"	28
Red Cabbage	"	7	"	28
Silverskin Onions	"	6	"	21
Sweet Pickle	"	40	"	143
Tomato & Chilli Relish	"	33	"	118
Tomato Relish	"	33	"	118
SAINSBURY				
Bread Sauce (made up)	1 tbs	30		
Brown Sauce	"	15		
Cheese Sauce (made up)	"	15		
Country Stuffing	1 oz	104	100 g	365
Curried Fruit Chutney	"	41	"	145
Fruit Sauce	1 tbs	20		
Horseradish	"	15		
Horseradish, creamed	"	45		
Mint Jelly	"	60		
Onion Sauce (made up)	"	15		
Parsley Sauce (made up)	"	15		
Salad Cream	"	110		
Tomato Sauce (Italian)	"	25		
Dressings				
Blue Cheese	1 fl. oz	149	100 g	525

Sauces, Pickles and Salad Dressings

Food	Quantities	Calories	Quantities	Calories
Garlic & Herb	1 fl. oz	92	100 g	325
Mild Curry	"	101	"	355
Reduced cal vinegar/oil	"	43	"	150
Thousand Island	"	43	"	150
Yoghurt & Chive	"	159	"	560
SPAR				
Mayonnaise	1 oz	213	100 g	750
WAITROSE				
Dressings				
Herb Cream	1 oz	64	100 g	224
Low Calorie Vinegar & Oil	"	43	"	150
Mayonnaise – all flavours	"	208	"	734
Salad Cream	"	92	"	324
1000 Island	"	55	"	194
Pickles				
Apple Chutney	"	55	"	193
Cocktail Gherkins	"	4	"	14
Cocktail Onions	"	8	"	27
Mango Chutney	"	63	"	221
Mixed Pickles	"	6	"	21
Piccalilli, Sweet	"	14	"	48
Pickled Baby Beetroots	"	7	"	26
Pickled Onions	"	5	"	19
Pickled Sweet Onions	"	11	"	38
Pickled Red Cabbage	"	6	"	21

Sauces, Pickles and Salad Dressings

Food	Quantities	Calories	Quantities	Calories
Pickled Sliced Beetroot	1 oz	10	100 g	37
Pickled Sliced Beetroot in Sweet Vinegar	”	16	”	55
Tomato Chutney	”	44	”	154
Pasta Sauces				
Arrabiata	”	9	”	33
Bolognese	”	20	”	70
Carbonara	”	57	”	200
Milanese	”	18	”	62
Napolitan	”	8	”	27
Siciliana	”	15	”	54
Stuffings				
Country Herb	”	91	”	320
Parsley, Thyme & Lemon	”	92	”	325
Sage & Onion	”	92	”	325
Other Sauces				
Creamed Horseradish	”	54	”	190
Fruit Sauce	”	34	”	120
Goulasch	”	23	”	80
Horseradish Sauce	”	23	”	80
Spicy Brown Sauce	”	38	”	98
Tartare Sauce	”	80	”	283
Tomato Ketchup	”	44	”	154

Savoury Spreads

Savoury Spreads made an excellent alternative 'packed lunch', as long as you don't eat too much bread or other starch with them. A sandwich made with savoury spread and plenty of salad is quite low in calories and very tasty.

Food	Quantities	Calories	Quantities	Calories
BOOTS				
Savoury Spread	1 oz	58	100 g	205
GRANOSE				
'Sandwich Spread'				
Cereals	1 oz	63	100 g	225
Herbs	”	74	”	263
Mushrooms	”	95	”	337
Olives	”	87	”	308
Soya Bean Paste	”	39	”	140
Tastex	”	59	”	208
Vegetable Paté	”	83	”	296

Food	Quantities	Calories	Quantities	Calories
HEINZ				
Spreads				
Celery, Corn & Apple	1 oz	53	100 g	188
Cucumber Sandwich	”	52	”	183
'Toast Toppers'				
Chicken & Mushroom	1 oz	15	”	54
Curried Chicken	”	21	”	73
Ham & Cheese	”	40	”	141
Mushroom & Bacon	”	37	”	131
Turkey and Ham	”	24	”	85
MARMITE	1 oz	50	1 tsp	13
MARKS & SPENCER				
Ham Spread	1 oz	55	100 g	193
Potted Beef	”	48	”	170
Potted Crab with Butter	”	51	”	180
Potted Salmon with Butter	”	47	”	166
Tuna Spread with Mayonnaise	”	93	”	329
NATEX				
Original Yeast Extract	1 oz	52	100 g	218
Low Salt Yeast Extract	”	52	”	218
PRINCES				
'Pastes'				
Beef	1 oz	60	100 g	212
Chicken & Ham	”	58	”	203

Savoury Spreads

Food	Quantities	Calories	Quantities	Calories
Crab	1 oz	39	100 g	139
Ham & Beef	,,	39	,,	139
Salmon	,,	29	,,	103
Sardine & Tomato	,,	43	,,	152
'Spreads'				
Beef	,,	56	,,	199
Crab Paté	,,	39	,,	138
Fried Chicken	,,	57	,,	201
Ham	,,	56	,,	196
Lobster Paté	,,	35	,,	125
Salmon Pate	,,	29	,,	101
Smokey Bacon	,,	61	,,	215
Tuna & Mayo Paté	,,	36	,,	126
'Toasties'				
Barbecued Chicken	,,	43	,,	152
Beef & Onion	,,	45	,,	159
Chicken & Sweetcorn	,,	49	,,	173
Ham & Cheese	,,	48	,,	170
Smokey Bacon	,,	57	,,	202
SAFEWAY				
Beef Paste	1 oz	64	100 g	225
Chicken & Ham Paste	,,	64	,,	225
Crab Paste	,,	53	,,	186
Salmon & Shrip	,,	52	,,	183
SHIPPAMS				
Anchovy Paste	35 g jar	60		

Food	Quantities	Calories	Quantities	Calories
Bacon/Beef/Liver Paste	35 g jar	70		
Bloater Paste	,,	65		
Chicken Spread	,,	80		
Chicken & Ham Spread	,,	75		
Crab Paste	,,	65		
Ham Spread	,,	60		
Salmon/Sardine & Tomato	,,	65		
Salmon & Shrip	,,	60		
'Country Pot'				
Anchovy	75 g jar	125		
Beef	,,	150		
Bloater	,,	135		
Chicken & Ham Spread	,,	155		
Ham & Beef	,,	140		
Liver & Bacon	,,	145		
Salmon & Shrimp	,,	130		

TARTEX
Original Yeast Spread	1 oz	65	100 g	229

VESSEN
Pate
Herb	1 pack	60		
Mushroom	,,	65		
Pepper	,,	50		

Soups

Soup is such a comforting and satisfying food if it is cold or if one is hungry. For remarkably few calories you can feel satisfied after a nice bowl of soup. There are so many good ones available and even the 'instant' variety, which you make in a cup, now comes in many flavours.

Food	Quantities	Calories	Quantities	Calories
BAXTERS				
Tinned				
Beef Consommé	1 oz	3	100 g	10
Chicken Broth	,,	10	,,	35
Cock-a-Leekie	,,	7	,,	25
Cream of Asparagus	,,	20	,,	70
Cream of Chicken	,,	18	,,	65
Cream of Leek	,,	14	,,	51
Cream of Mushroom	,,	15	,,	54
Cream of Pheasant	,,	17	,,	60
Cream of Scampi	,,	16	,,	57

Food	Quantities	Calories	Quantities	Calories
Cream of Smoked Trout	1 oz	15	100 g	55
Cream of Tomato	”	20	”	72
French Onion	”	8	”	28
Game Consommé	”	2	”	9
Highlander's Broth	”	13	”	47
Lentil	”	15	”	54
Lobster Bisque	”	19	”	67
Minestrone	”	10	”	37
Oxtail	”	13	”	47
Pea & Ham	”	13	”	47
Poacher's Broth	”	11	”	41
Royal Game	”	11	”	41
Scotch Salmon Bisque	”	22	”	78
Scotch Broth	”	13	”	48
Scotch Vegetable	”	9	”	29

BONNE CUISINE
Packet – dry

Food	Quantities	Calories	Quantities	Calories
Cream of Asparagus	1 oz	93	100 g	329
Cream of Chicken	”	93	”	327
Cream of Mushroom	”	91	”	320
Cream of Vegetable	”	92	”	324
Game	”	59	”	208
Lobster Bisque	”	76	”	268

BOOTS
'Second Nature' *(dry)*

Food	Quantities	Calories	Quantities	Calories
Green Rye with Mushroom	1 oz	91	100 g	319

Soups

Food	Quantities	Calories	Quantities	Calories
Mixed Vegetable & Spice	1 oz	96	100 g	338
Thick Green Bean	"	90	"	313
Thick Potato	"	89	"	313
CAMPBELL'S *(tinned)*				
'Bumper Harvest'				
Chicken	1 oz	12	100 g	44
Lentil	"	13	"	45
Mushroom	"	12	"	42
Minestrone	"	12	"	43
Oxtail	"	12	"	44
Pea	"	16	"	55
Scotch Broth	"	11	"	40
Tomato	"	17	"	59
Vegetable	"	11	"	40
'Condensed'				
Asparagus	"	9	"	31
Beef Broth	"	10	"	34
Chicken, Cream of	"	14	"	49
Chicken Noodle	"	5	"	18
Chicken Rice	"	7	"	25
Chicken & Sweetcorn	"	12	"	44
Celery, Cream of	"	12	"	41
Consommé	"	1	"	4
Crab Bisque	"	10	"	37
French Onion	"	4	"	15
Golden Vegetable	"	7	"	24

Food	Quantities	Calories	Quantities	Calories
Goulash	1 oz	12	100 g	43
Lentil	,,	12	,,	44
Oxtail	,,	12	,,	43
Pea & Ham	,,	18	,,	62
Scotch Broth	,,	10	,,	36
Smoked Salmon, Cream of	,,	15	,,	53
Tomato	,,	9	,,	33
Tomato, Cream of	,,	18	,,	62
Tomato Rice	,,	14	,,	48
Turkey & Veg Broth	,,	11	,,	38
'Main Course'				
Beef & Vegetables	,,	16	,,	55
Chicken & Vegetables	,,	14	,,	51
Steak, Kidney & Veg	,,	16	,,	55
'Granny'				
Chicken	,,	11	,,	40
Chicken & Veg. Broth	,,	7	,,	25
Lentil	,,	10	,,	37
Pea & Ham	,,	10	,,	35
Potato Leek	,,	8	,,	29
Scotch Broth	,,	10	,,	37
Tomato	,,	8	,,	27
Vegetable	,,	7	,,	26
Veg. Broth with Beef	,,	6	,,	23
CROSSE & BLACKWELL *(tinned)*				
Chicken, Cream of	1 oz	18	100 g	63

Soups

Food	Quantities	Calories	Quantities	Calories
Consommé	1 oz	6	100 g	22
Country Vegetable with Beef	,,	12	,,	41
Creamed Tomato	,,	20	,,	71
Creamed Tomato				
Herbs	,,	21	,,	73
Mint	,,	20	,,	70
Onion & Pepper	,,	21	,,	71
Spices	,,	20	,,	71
Farmhouse Thick Vegetable	,,	15	,,	53
Minestrone	,,	14	,,	48
Mushroom, Cream of	,,	15	,,	54
Oxtail	,,	14	,,	49
Oxtail & Vegetable	,,	11	,,	38
Scotch Broth	,,	18	,,	62
Scottish Lentil with Veg.	,,	13	,,	45
Spanish Style & Sweet Pepper	,,	13	,,	45
Vegetable	,,	14	,,	48
Vichyssoise	,,	13	,,	47
'Chef Chunky'				
Chicken	,,	12	,,	44
Tomato & Vegetable	,,	10	,,	37
Vegetable	,,	12	,,	41
Vegetable & Beef	,,	12	,,	41
'Box Soups' (reconstituted)				
Beef Flavour with Veg	,,	7	,,	25
Chicken & Leek	,,	8	,,	27
Chicken Noodle	,,	7	,,	26

Food	Quantities	Calories	Quantities	Calories
Golden Vegetable	1 oz	8	100 g	29
Minestrone	''	8	''	28
Mushroom	''	8	''	28
Oxtail	''	8	''	29
Pea with Ham	''	8	''	29
Spring Vegetable	''	4	''	16
Thick Chicken	''	8	''	30
Thick Country Vegetable	''	9	''	32
Thick Garden Vegetable	''	7	''	25
Thick Onion	''	8	''	29
Thick Pea	''	7	''	26
Tomato	''	10	''	36
'Pot Soup Range'				
Country Chicken & Leek	1 sachet	62		
Farmhouse Potato & Veg.	''	65		
Harvest Veg. & Beef	''	74		
Rich Tomato	''	78		
HEINZ 'Big Soups'				
Beef and Vegetable	1 oz	10	100 g	36
Beef Broth	''	8	''	29
Chicken & Vegetable	''	10	''	37
Golden Vegetable	''	12	''	41
Vegetable	''	11	''	39
'Classic Soups'				
Cream of Asparagus	''	12	''	43

Soups

Food	Quantities	Calories	Quantities	Calories
Cream of Chicken with White Wine	1 oz	14	100 g	50
Cock-a-Leekie	"	6	"	20
Mild Creamy Curried Chicken	"	15	"	52
Rich Oxtail with Sherry	"	10	"	35
Special Cream of Mushroom	"	11	"	40
'Ready to Serve Soups'				
Beef Broth	"	11	"	39
Beef Soup	"	10	"	37
Cream of Celery	"	12	"	43
Cream of Chicken	"	13	"	46
Farmhouse Thick Vegetable	"	14	"	48
Golden Chicken and Mushroom	"	12	"	42
Golden Chicken and Vegetable	"	10	"	34
Golden Vegetable	"	12	"	41
Homestyle Beef & Vegetable	"	11	"	39
Homestyle Country Vegetable	"	12	"	43
Homestyle Potato & Leek	"	10	"	36
Invaders	"	20	"	71
Lentil	"	10	"	35
Minestrone	"	9	"	31
Mulligatawny	"	14	"	48
Mushroom	"	13	"	45

Food	Quantities	Calories	Quantities	Calories
Oxtail	1 oz	16	100 g	56
Pea & Ham	"	16	"	56
Scotch Broth	"	12	"	43
Scottish Vegetable with Lentils	"	9	"	33
Spring Vegetable	"	17	"	60
Tomato	"	10	"	37
Vegetable	"	10	"	37
HERA *(dry)*				
Farmhouse Vegetable	25 g	94	100 g	376
Minestrone	"	96	"	382
Tomato	"	91	"	364
Vegetable Goulash	"	94	"	376
HOLLAND & BARRETT *(dry)*				
Soup Mixes	1 oz	81	100 g	285
KNORR *(dry)*				
Chicken Noodle	1 packet	187	100 g	347
Cornish Seafood	"	278	"	374
Crofters' Thick Vegetable	"	242	"	310
Farmhouse Chicken & Leek	"	233	"	338
Florida Spring Vegetable	"	106	"	280
Highland Lentil	"	301	"	314
Minestrone	"	243	"	312
Oxtail	"	250	"	327

Soups

Food	Quantities	Calories	Quantities	Calories
Pea with Ham	1 packet	206	100 g	327
Virginia Sweetcorn	"	328	"	368
'Blended Soups'				
Country Vegetable	"	222	"	337
Golden Vegetable	"	241	"	340
Tomato & Vegetable	"	213	"	300
Vegetable & Leek	"	219	"	313
'No Simmer Cream Soups'				
Asparagus	"	363	"	497
Chicken	"	390	"	500
Mushroom	"	373	"	484
Tomato	"	418	"	459
'Quick Soups'				
Chicken	"	86	"	420
Chicken & Leek	"	85	"	414
Chicken & Mushroom	"	75	"	403
Golden Vegetable	"	83	"	427
Oxtail	"	62	"	363
Pea with Ham	"	67	"	354
Tomato	"	95	"	395
'Light Drinks'				
Beef	1 cup	21		
Chicken	"	22		
Vegetable	"	20		
MARKS & SPENCER (tinned)				
Beef & Vegetable	1 oz	21	100 g	76

Food	Quantities	Calories	Quantities	Calories
Chicken & Vegetable	1 oz	16	100 g	58
Cream of Tomato	”	16	”	55
Cream of Asparagus	”	18	”	64
Cream of Smoked Trout	”	18	”	64
Lobster Bisque	”	15	”	52
Mediterranean Vegetable	”	10	”	37
Pea & Ham	”	17	”	60
PREWETT'S				
'Easy Cook'				
Lincoln Pea	1 pkt	77	100 g	308
Mushroom	”	83	”	330
Tomato	”	82	”	326
'In Seconds'				
Lentil	”	59	”	296
Mushroom	”	60	”	302
Tomato	”	65	”	313
SAFEWAY *(dry)*				
Asparagus	1 oz	104	100 g	366
Chicken Noodle	”	80	”	283
Golden Vegetable	”	87	”	308
Minestrone	”	79	”	280
Mushroom	”	135	”	477
Oxtail	”	89	”	315
Spring Vegetable	”	68	”	238
Thick Chicken	”	141	”	495

Soups

Food	Quantities	Calories	Quantities	Calories
Tomato	1 oz	91	100 g	320
'Instant' (dry)				
Beef & Tomato	"	100	"	354
Chicken	"	112	"	395
Golden Vegetable	"	103	"	363
Mushroom	"	98	"	347
Tomato	"	96	"	338
(Instant with croutons) (dry)				
Asparagus	"	132	"	464
Chicken & Vegetable	"	107	"	376
French Onion	"	114	"	400
Minestrone	"	104	"	365
(tinned)				
Celery, Cream of	1 fl. oz	15	100 ml	52
Chicken, Cream of	"	16	"	56
Lentil	"	11	"	40
Mushroom, Cream of	"	19	"	68
Oxtail	"	12	"	42
Pea & Ham	"	16	"	58
Scotch Broth	"	12	"	43
Tomato, Cream of	"	19	"	66
Vegetable	"	11	"	39
SAINSBURY				
'Soup In A Cup' (dry)				
Bacon & Tomato	1 oz	108	100 g	380
Chicken & Mushroom	"	114	"	400

Food	Quantities	Calories	Quantities	Calories
Chicken & Vegetable	1 oz	109	100 g	385
Minestrone	”	96	”	340
Tomato & Vegetable	”	98	”	345
(tinned)				
Asparagus, Cream of	½ pint	165	100 ml	55
Chicken, Cream of	”	180	”	60
Consomme	”	45	”	15
Crab Bisque	”	135	”	45
Extra Thick Vegetable	”	150	”	50
French Onion	”	75	”	25
Lobster Bisque	”	180	”	60
Minestrone	”	135	”	45
Oxtail	”	150	”	50
Scotch Broth	”	165	”	55
Tomato, Cream of	”	225	”	75
Tuna & Sweetcorn	”	135	”	45
Vegetable	”	135	”	45
Vegetable & Beef	”	195	”	65
Vichyssoise	”	135	”	45
(Packet, reconstituted)				
Asparagus	”	132	”	44
Beef & Tomato	”	67	”	23
Chicken	”	110	”	37
Chicken & Leek	”	82	”	28
Chicken Noodle	”	85	”	28
French Onion	”	42	”	14
Golden Vegetable	”	97	”	35

Soups

Food	Quantities	Calories	Quantities	Calories
Minestrone	½ pint	67	100 ml	22
Mushroom	”	85	”	28
Onion	”	82	”	28
Spring Vegetable	”	67	”	22
Tomato	”	95	”	32
Vegetable	”	95	”	32
Vegetable & Beef	”	92	”	31
'Soup A Snack' *(dry)*				
Pasta, Chicken & Mushroom	1 oz	114	100 g	400
Pasta, Tomato & Vegetable	”	99	”	350
Pasta, Vegetable & Beef	”	99	”	350
'Soup In A Cup' *(dry)*				
Asparagus	”	102	”	360
Chicken	”	105	”	370
Chicken & Leek	”	105	”	370
French Onion	”	89	”	315
Golden Vegetable	”	99	”	350
Mushroom	”	105	”	370
Sweetcorn & Chicken	”	104	”	365
Tomato	”	99	”	350
Tomato & Beef	”	96	”	340
WAITROSE *(tinned)*				
Asparagus, Cream of	1 fl. oz	16	100 ml	55
Beef Broth	”	11	”	40
Celery, Cream of	”	15	”	54
Chicken, Cream of	”	16	”	58

Food	Quantities	Calories	Quantities	Calories
Clam Chowder	1 fl. oz	12	100 ml	43
Cock-a-Leekie	,,	7	,,	24
Cornish Crab Bisque	,,	22	,,	78
French Onion	,,	4	,,	15
Lentil Soup	,,	14	,,	49
Lobster Bisque	,,	14	,,	51
Minestrone	,,	13	,,	47
Mushroom, Cream of	,,	15	,,	53
Pea & Ham	,,	16	,,	56
Oxtail	,,	11	,,	38
Scotch Broth	,,	10	,,	37
Tomato, Cream of	,,	18	,,	63
Vegetable	,,	12	,,	44
Vichyssoise	,,	15	,,	54
(Packet – *dry*)				
Asparagus	,,	93	,,	326
Chicken	,,	81	,,	287
Chicken & Leek	,,	107	,,	376
Chicken Noodle	,,	86	,,	303
French Onion	,,	89	,,	315
Minestrone	,,	87	,,	307
Mushroom	,,	96	,,	340
Spring Vegetable	,,	81	,,	286

Sweets & Chocolates

It could be argued that this section should not be in this book at all, that people who have to count calories should not even consider sweets or chocolates. This is unrealistic as there is hardly a person alive who doesn't occasionally crave something sweet, probably chocolate! So there is definitely a place for these products in this book so that the calories already consumed, or about to be consumed, may be accurately counted.

Food	Quantities	Calories	Quantities	Calories
BOOTS				
Non-chocolate				
Acid Drops	1 oz	103	100 g	363
Aniseed Drops	"	103	"	363
Apple Drops	"	103	"	363
Barley Sugar Drops	"	103	"	363
Bitter Lemon Drops	"	103	"	363

Food	Quantities	Calories	Quantities	Calories
Blackcurrant Drops				
with Vit. C	1 oz	103	100 g	363
Butter Drops	”	127	”	448
Fruit Flavour Drops	”	103	”	363
Fresh Mints	”	103	”	363
Golden Mints	”	103	”	363
Lemon & Lime Drops	”	103	”	363
Liquorice Drops	”	127	”	448
Mint Humbugs	”	105	”	371
Mixed Fruit Drops	”	103	”	363
Old Fashioned Mixture Drops	”	103	”	363
'Soft Pastilles'				
Glycerin, Honey,				
Blackcurrant	”	91	”	322
Glycerin, Honey, Lemon	”	90	”	318
Glycerine, Honey, Orange	”	90	”	318
'Stick Packs'				
Honey Menthol	”	103	”	363
Menthol-Eucalyptus	”	103	”	363
Menthol Mints	”	103	”	363
CADBURY				
Bar Six	1 bar	220	100 g	550
Boost	”	255	”	485
Bournville Dark	1 oz	145	”	510
Brazil Nut	”	156	”	550
Butter Mints	each	30	”	435

Sweets & Chocolates

Food	Quantities	Calories	Quantities	Calories
Buttons	large pkt	270	”	530
Buttons	standard pkt	175		
Caramel	”	245	”	490
Chocolate Cream	”	210	”	420
Crunchie	small	110	”	465
Crunchie	standard	195		
Curly Wurly	one	135	”	470
Dairy Milk	1 oz	150	”	530
Dairy Milk Miniatures	each	30	”	530
Double Decker	one bar	235	”	465
Five Centre	”	215	”	425
Flake	”	180	”	530
Flake 99	”	65	”	530
Fruit & Nut	1 oz	133	”	470
Fudge	1 bar	130	”	435
Fresh Mints	each	25		
Fruit Bonbons	pocket pack	20	”	380
Gambit	1 bar	210	”	520
Milk Chocolate Eclairs	pocket pack	20	”	450
Murray Fruits	each	25	”	390
Murray Mints	pocket pack	25	”	400
Picnic	each	230	”	495
Peppermint Cream	”	210	”	420
Roast Almond	”	153	”	540
Shortcake Snack	1 biscuit	35	”	490
Skippy	each	190	”	455
Star Bar	”	260	”	495

Food	Quantities	Calories	Quantities	Calories
Sultana	each	128	"	450
Turkish Delight	"	185	"	360
Wholenut	1 oz	158	"	555
Wispa	each	200	"	565

FERRERO

Food	Quantities	Calories	Quantities	Calories
Ferrero Rocher	1 oz	166	100 g	585
Kinder Chocolate	"	160	"	565
Kinder Friends	"	168	"	590
Mon Cheri	"	121	"	428
Opera Liqueur Chocolates	"	107	"	378
Tic Tac	each	2		

FOX'S

Food	Quantities	Calories
Glacier Fruits – stick pack	1 sweet	10
Glacier Fruits – bag	"	20
Glacier Mints – stick pack	"	10
Glacier Mints – bag	"	20

FRY'S

Food	Quantities	Calories
Chocolate Cream	1 bar	210
Five Centres	"	215
Peppermint Cream	"	210
Turkish Delight	"	185

KEILLER

Food	Quantities	Calories	Quantities	Calories
Butterscotch	1 oz	110	100 g	387

Sweets & Chocolates

Food	Quantities	Calories	Quantities	Calories
Mint Butterscotch	1 oz	110	100 g	387
LUCOZADE				
Glucose Energy Tablets	each	10		
MARKS & SPENCER				
Chocolate				
Birds Eggs, milk chocolate	1 oz	122	100 g	430
Bubbly Bar	”	157	”	552
Buttons, Milk Chocolate	”	141	”	496
Caramel Ministicks	”	134	”	473
Champagne Truffles	”	166	”	584
Chocolate Ginger	”	114	”	400
Cocktail Chocolates	”	136	”	479
Cointreau Sticks	”	119	”	420
Crunch	”	128	”	450
Drops, Milk Chocolate	”	122	”	430
Fresh Cream Chocolate Truffles	”	142		536
Fresh Cream Liqueur Truffles	”	148	”	522
Fudge Bars	”	127	”	447
Hazelnut Ministicks	”	156	”	550
Honeycomb Crunch	”	128	”	450
Irresistibles				
Marzipan/Praline	”	154	”	542
Praline	”	128	”	450

Food	Quantities	Calories	Quantities	Calories
Praline & Wafer	1 oz	148	100 g	523
Liqueur Truffles	"	147	"	519
Milk Chocolate	"	152	"	535
Milk Chocolate with Strawberries	"	162	"	572
Milk Chocolate with Caramel	"	126	"	445
Milk Chocolate Mini Sticks	"	150	"	528
Milk Chocolate Eclairs	"	123	"	432
Milk Chocolate Caramels/ Fudge	"	129	"	455
Milk Chocolate Peanut Cracknel	"	125	"	440
Mints, Chocolate	"	115	"	406
Mocca Mini Sticks	"	157	"	554
Noisettes	"	150	"	527
Plain Chocolate	"	151	"	531
Royale Truffles	"	162	"	571
Swiss Mountain Bar	"	156	"	550
Swiss Mountain Bar – White	"	151	"	562
Take 4	"	143	"	502
Walnut Whips	"	135	"	474
Non-chocolate				
Butter Fudge	"	68	"	240
Butter Mintoes	"	116	"	410
Buttermints	"	108	"	381
Butter Toffee Assortment	"	124	"	437
Crystal Fruit Drops	"	102	"	358

Sweets & Chocolates

Food	Quantities	Calories	Quantities	Calories
Fruit Chews	1 oz	105	100 g	370
Fruit Pastilles Assorted	"	.98	"	344
Jelly Babies	"	92	"	323
Liquorice Allsorts	"	104	"	368
Liquorice Sandwiches	"	98	"	346
Marzipan Fruits	"	122	"	429
Mint Assortment	"	106	"	375
Real Fruit Gums	"	96	"	340
Sherbert Fruit Flavoured	"	89	"	313
Soft Gum Animals	"	83	"	292
Soft & Smooth Caramels	"	138	"	485
Sugared Almonds	"	131	"	460
Teddy Bear Gums	"	96	"	340
Vanilla Toffee	"	154	"	542
Wine Gums	"	97	"	342

MARS
Chocolate

Food	Quantities	Calories
Bounty milk	1 bar	280
Bounty Plain	"	281
Bounty	funsize	140
Galaxy	50 g	273
Maltesers	standard	191
Maltesers	funsize	111
Marathon	1 bar	315
Marathon	funsize	98
Mars Bar	1 bar	295

Food	Quantities	Calories	Quantities	Calories
Mars Bar	funsize	88		
Milky Way	1 bar	130		
Milky Way	funsize	73		
Minstrels	1 pack	244		
Revels	standard	176		
Ripple	1 bar	171		
Topic	,,	248		
Tracker, choc. chip	1 bar	202		
Tracker, roast nut	,,	202		
Treets	standard	235		
Twix	1 bar	300		
Twix	teabreak	150		
Non-chocolate				
Lockets	1 pack	153		
Opals	51 g pack	199		
Skittles	50 g pack	187		
Tunes	1 pack	136		
MAYNARD				
American Hard Gums	1 bag	415		
Chocolate Coconut Ice	1 bar	360		
Chocolate Mint Coconut Ice	,,	365		
Chocolate Limes	,,	365		
Empress Mixture	,,	360		
Jelly Beans	,,	375		
Milk Gums	,,	330		
Mint Imperials	,,	420		

Sweets & Chocolates

Food	Quantities	Calories	Quantities	Calories
Misty	1 bar	170		
Nougat	"	185		
Nougat, soft	small bar	110		
Whipped Bon Bons	1 bag	440		
Wine Gums	"	355		
NESTLES				
Fruit & Nut Chocolate	1 oz	135	100 g	475
Milk Chocolate	"	152	"	534
Milky Bar	"	153	"	534
Plain Superfine	"	155	"	546
Whole Nut	"	158	"	557
ROWNTREE MACKINTOSH				
Chocolate				
Aero	1 oz	148	100 g	521
Aero, orange	"	149	"	527
Aero, peppermint	"	151	"	532
After Eight	"	116	"	409
Black Magic	"	126	"	444
Cabana	"	125	"	440
Caramac	"	157	"	553
Dairy Box	"	126	"	444
Drifter	"	76	"	261
Golden Cup				
large	"	133	"	467
medium	"	131	"	461

Food	Quantities	Calories	Quantities	Calories
small	1 oz	129	100 g	455
Kit Kat	,,	143	,,	500
Lion Bar	,,	141	,,	496
Matchmakers				
coffee	,,	135	,,	477
orange	,,	136	,,	478
peppermint	,,	136	,,	480
Mintola	,,	124	,,	437
Minty Egg	,,	118	,,	415
Munchies	,,	140	,,	494
Novo	,,	121	,,	428
Quality Street	,,	129	,,	455
Rolo	,,	127	,,	447
Savana	,,	136	,,	478
Smarties	,,	129	,,	455
Toffee Crisp	,,	144	,,	507
Walnut Whips	,,	139	,,	489
Yorkie				
milk	,,	145	,,	510
almond	,,	150	,,	528
hazelnut & orange	,,	136	,,	478
raisin & biscuit	,,	161	,,	460
Non-chocolate				
Fruit Gums	,,	79	,,	278
Fruit Pastilles	,,	93	,,	329
Glace Fruits	,,	104	,,	368
Glace Mints	,,	105	,,	371

Sweets & Chocolates

Food	Quantities	Calories	Quantities	Calories
Polo Fruits	1 oz	105	100 g	370
Polo Mints	''	107	''	377
Toffee, Assorted	''	133	''	468
Toffee, Golden	''	130	''	457
Toffo				
Assorted/Mint	''	129	''	454
Plain	''	128	''	451
Tootie Frooties	''	112	''	394
Tooty Minties	''	112	''	396
Tots				
Bunny	''	120	''	422
Candy	''	110	''	388
Jelly	''	97	''	341
Tiger	''	109	''	384
SAFEWAY				
Funtime Fudge Bars	1 oz	127	100 g	447
Funtime Honeycomb Crunch	''	128	''	450
Honeycomb Crunch Bars	''	128	''	450
Milk Chocolate Brazils	''	157	''	554
Milk Chocolate Buttons	''	139	''	490
Plain Chocolate Brazils	''	156	''	551
Sugared Almonds	''	130	''	458
SPAR				
Non-chocolate				
American Hard Gums	1 oz	97	100 g	342

Food	Quantities	Calories	Quantities	Calories
Barley Sugar	1 oz	110	100 g	387
Brazil Nut Toffee	,,	124	,,	437
Butterscotch	,,	121	,,	425
Chewy Fruits	,,	78	,,	275
Chewy Sherbet Fruits	,,	75	,,	263
Chocolate Flavoured Eclairs	,,	123	,,	432
Clear Fruit Drops	,,	102	,,	358
Coconut Toasties	,,	88	,,	309
Devon Toffee	,,	103	,,	364
Dolly Mixtures	,,	104	,,	366
Dusted Jelly Babies	,,	88	,,	311
Extra Strong Mints	,,	.90	,,	316
Fruit & Nut Nougat	,,	88	,,	309
Fruit Jellies	,,	85	,,	300
Fruit Pastilles	,,	91	,,	322
Jelly Drops	,,	85	,,	300
Liquorice Allsorts	,,	97	,,	342
Liquorice Cuttings	,,	82	,,	289
Marshmallow	,,	87	,,	303
Mint Humbugs	,,	108	,,	379
Mint Imperials	,,	105	,,	371
Mintoes	,,	116	,,	409
Nut Brittle	,,	99	,,	350
Nutty Toffee Puffs	,,	125	,,	440
Sherbet Fruits	,,	81	,,	285
Sparkling Mints	,,	106	,,	374
Sugared Tea Cakes	,,	96	,,	337

Sweets & Chocolates

Food	Quantities	Calories	Quantities	Calories
Toffee Assortment	1 oz	103	100 g	364
Toffee Popcorn	"	108	"	381
Vanilla Fudge	"	114	"	398
Wine Gums	"	92	"	324
Chocolate				
Chewing Nuts	"	86	"	304
Peanuts	"	158	"	552
Raisins	"	106	"	373
WAITROSE				
Butter Mintoes	1 oz	112	100 g	396
Clear Fruits	"	102	"	358
Clear Mints	"	102	"	360
Devon Toffees	"	122	"	430
Fruit Jellies	"	84	"	296
Fruit Pastilles	"	91	"	322
Imperial Mints	"	105	"	377
Jelly Animals	"	88	"	311
Liquorice Allsorts	"	104	"	368
Mint Assortment	"	107	"	377
Mint Humbugs	"	103	"	362
Wine Gums	"	97	"	342
Chocolate				
Chocolate Brazils	"	163	"	574
Chocolate Ginger	"	109	"	384
Chocolate Peppermint Creams	"	118	"	414

Sweets & Chocolates

Food	Quantities	Calories	Quantities	Calories
Mint Crisp Chocolates	1 oz	139	100 g	489
Plain Chocolate	”	150	”	530
Plain Chocolate with Hazelnuts	”	157	”	554

Vegetables & Pulses

Vegetable are – with a few exceptions – virtually calorie-free and should be eaten in large quantities by anybody on a slimming diet. The problem is that they taste so much better when served with lots of butter and *that* is when the calories appear. To make them taste good it is most important not to overcook them. Lemon juice and soy sauce are both useful additions instead of butter. It is now being said that frozen vegetables have more goodness than some of the so-called 'fresh' vegetables found in supermarkets as the latter have frequently been on the road from field to shop for quite some time.

Food	Quantities	Calories	Quantities	Calories
BEJAM *(frozen)*				
Baby Carrots	1 oz	6	100 g	21
Battered Onion Rings	"	106	"	373
Brussels Sprouts	"	13	"	46

Food	Quantities	Calories	Quantities	Calories
Button Sprouts	1 oz	13	100 g	46
Broad Beans	"	25	"	88
Broccoli Spears	"	7	"	25
Cabbage, Cut	"	7	"	25
Cauliflower Florets	"	5	"	18
Chilli Bean Mix	"	30	"	106
Continental Mix	"	10	"	35
Corn-on-the-Cob	7 oz cob	165		
Courgettes, slices	"	18	"	63
Crisp Crumb Cauliflower Florets	"	48	"	169
Economy Garden Peas	"	26	"	91
Farmhouse Style Mix	"	6	"	21
Fine Whole Beans	"	10	"	35
Fluted Carrot Rings	"	6	"	21
Green Beans, Cut	"	7	"	25
Green Beans, Sliced	"	9	"	32
Grean Beans, Whole	"	9	"	32
Leeks, Creamed	1 mini portion	10		
Leeks, Cut	1 oz	7	"	25
Mange Touts	"	13	"	46
Mexican Mix	"	16	"	56
Mini Corn Cobs	2 mini cobs	174		
Minted Garden Peas	"	19	"	69
Mixed Vegetables	"	17	"	60
Mushrooms, Sliced	"	3	"	10
Mushrooms, Whole	"	4	"	14

Vegetables & Pulses

Food	Quantities	Calories	Quantities	Calories
Onions, Sliced	1 oz	3	100 g	10
Onions, Small Whole	"	11	"	39
Oriental Mix	"	9	"	32
Parsnips, Small Whole	"	19	"	67
Pasta Mix	"	19	"	67
Peas, Grade A	"	22	"	77
Peppers, Sliced Mixed	"	8	"	28
Petits Pois	"	22	"	77
Petits Pois & Baby Carrots	"	11	"	39
'Potato Products'				
American Fries (fried)	6 oz portion	402		
Crinkle Cut Chips (fried)	"	300		
Crinkle Cut Oven Chips (baked)	"	237		
Crispy Potato Waffles	each	95		
Oven Steak Chips (baked)	6 oz portion	214		
Potato Croquettes (fried)	each	41		
Potato Pancakes (grilled)	"	97		
Steak Fries (fried)	6 oz portion	255		
Straight Cut Oven Chips (baked)	"	227		
Red Cabbage with Apple	1 mini portion	10	"	49
Ratatouille	1 oz	14	"	49
Special Chinese Vegetables	"	8	"	28
Spinach,				
Chopped	"	6	"	21
Creamed	1 mini portion	11		

Food	Quantities	Calories	Quantities	Calories
Leaf	1 oz	7	"	25
Spring Vegetable Mix	"	10	"	35
Stewpack	"	5	"	18
Swede, Diced	"	6	"	21
Sweetcorn	"	31	"	109
Veg 'n' Rice Mix	"	13	"	46
BIRD'S EYE				
Alphabites				
grilled	1 oz	60	100 g	211
deep fried	"	65	"	229
shallow fried	"	85	"	299
Baby Broad Beans	"	15	"	53
Baby Carrots	"	5	"	18
Bacon & Cheese				
Jacket Potatoes	½ potato	190		
Broccoli Mornay	1 oz	31	"	110
Broccoli Spears	"	7	"	25
Brussels Sprouts	"	10	"	35
Casserole Vegetables	"	10	"	35
Cauliflower	"	5	"	18
Cauliflower, Peas & Carrots	"	10	"	32
Cheese & Onion				
Jacket Potatoes	½	190		
Chips				
deep fried	1 oz	70	"	246
shallow fried	"	65	"	229

Vegetables & Pulses

Food	Quantities	Calories	Quantities	Calories
Chopped Cabbage	1 oz	6	100 g	21
Corn on the Cob	"	20	"	70
Country Club Jacket Peas	"	12	"	42
Country Potato Bake	1 pkt	435		
Crispy Potato Fritters	1 oz	60	"	211
Croquette Potatoes	one	5	"	20
Crunchy Potato Grill	1 oz	60	"	211
Original Mixed Vegetables	"	15	"	53
Oven Chips	"	55	"	194
Oven Stars				
grilled	"	65	"	229
fried	"	85	"	299
Peas	"	15	"	53
Peas & Baby Carrots	"	10	"	35
Petits Pois, Button Sprouts &				
Baby Carrots	"	12	"	42
Potato Waffles				
baked or grilled	one	115		
fried	"	175		
Potato Waffles, Mini				
baked or grilled	"	22		
fried	"	27		
Ratatouille	1 oz	17	"	60
Rice, Peas & Mushroom	"	35	"	123
Rice, Sweetcorn, Peas				
& Carrots	"	35	"	123
Sliced Green Beans	"	8	"	28

Food	Quantities	Calories	Quantities	Calories
Spinach, Leaf	1 oz	5	100 g	18
'Stir Fried' as sold				
Continental	,,	12	,,	42
Country	,,	8	,,	28
Oriental	,,	20	,,	70
Sweetcorn	,,	30	,,	106
Sweet Corn, Peas & Carrots	,,	15	,,	53
Vegetable Pasta	,,	40	,,	141
Whole Green Beans	,,	10	,,	35
BOOTS				
Borlotti Beans	1 oz	30	100 g	105
Butter Beans	,,	27	,,	95
Chick Peas	,,	23	,,	85
Haricot Beans	,,	27	,,	95
Red Kidney Beans	,,	31	,,	109
BUITONI				
Ratatouille	1 oz	10	100 g	37
Tomato Puree	,,	20	,,	72
CADURY				
Smash (dry)	1 oz	55	100 g	265
FINDUS *(frozen)*				
Broad Beans	1 oz	15	100 g	53
Broccoli Spears	,,	9	,,	32

Vegetables & Pulses

Food	Quantities	Calories	Quantities	Calories
Brussels Sprouts	1 oz	7	100 g	26
Cauliflower Fleurettes	”	4	”	13
Chips	”	31	”	109
Corn-on-the-Cob	”	36	”	127
Country Mix	”	16	”	55
Green Beans, Sliced	”	8	”	30
Haricot Verts	”	19	”	67
Mixed Vegetables	”	18	”	59
Peas	”	15	”	53
Petits Pois	”	18	”	63
Potato Croquettes	”	26	”	91
Potato Cakes, Swiss Style	”	23	”	80
Potatoes, saute	”	27	”	97
Spinach, chopped	”	9	”	32
Spinach, whole leaf	”	9	”	32
Summer Harvest Mix	”	20	”	72

HOLLAND & BARRETT

Food	Quantities	Calories	Quantities	Calories
Adzuki Beans	1 oz	68	100 g	238
Mung Beans	”	66	”	231
Red Kidney Beans	”	77	”	272
Soya Beans	”	114	”	400

MARKS & SPENCER

Food	Quantities	Calories	Quantities	Calories
Baked Bean Jackets	1 oz	34	100 g	120
Broccoli in Cream Sauce	”	26	”	93
Cabbage & Mushroom Bake	”	30	”	107

Food	Quantities	Calories	Quantities	Calories
Cauliflower Cheese	1 oz	42	100 g	149
Chinese Style Rice	"	43	"	151
Crispy Mushrooms	"	46	"	162
Filled Green Pepper	"	27	"	95
Fresh Vegetable Dip	"	204	"	718
Garden Vegetable Pie	"	32	"	113
Leek & Carrot Jacket Potato	"	43	"	151
Leek & Ham Bake	"	29	"	104
Mushroom Jacket Potato	"	43	"	153
Onion Bhajjis	"	60	"	211
Pancakes Mushroom/Beer Batter	"	48	"	171
Potato Bake	"	45	"	158
Potato Croquettes	"	43	"	151
Ratatouille	"	18	"	63

ROSS *(frozen)*

Food	Quantities	Calories	Quantities	Calories
Broad Beans	1 oz	16	100 g	55
Broccoli Mix	"	11	"	40
Broccoli Spears	"	6	"	20
Brussels Sprouts	"	8	"	30
Carrots	"	6	"	20
Cauliflower Florets	"	6	"	20
Casserole Mix	"	6	"	20
Country Mix	"	8	"	30
Farmhouse Mixed Vegetables	"	8	"	30
French Vegetable Mix	"	7	"	25

Vegetables & Pulses

Food	Quantities	Calories	Quantities	Calories
Green Beans	1 oz	7	100 g	25
Japanese Stir Fry	"	20	"	70
Leaf Spinach	"	8	"	30
Mexican Stir-Fry	"	19	"	31
Mixed Peppers	"	6	"	20
Onion Ringers	"	65	"	230
Oriental Vegetable Mix	"	11	"	40
Peas	"	6	"	14
'Potato Products'				
Bubble & Squeak	"	17	"	60
Chip Shop Chips	"	25	"	70
Chunky Chips	"	35	"	100
Crinkle Cut Chips	"	46	"	130
Crisp Crosses	"	51	"	180
Croquettes	"	28	"	100
Duchesse	"	31	"	110
French Fries	"	34	"	120
Hash Browns	"	20	"	70
Jacket Scallops	"	28	"	100
Jacket Wedges	"	34	"	120
Oven Chips	"	40	"	140
Oven Crunches	"	45	"	160
Pancakes	"	60	"	210
Roast Potatoes	"	28	"	100
Straight Cut Chips	"	31	"	110
Waffles	"	54	"	190
Ratatouille Mix	"	4	"	15

Vegetables & Pulses

Food	Quantities	Calories	Quantities	Calories
Shredded Cabbage	1 oz	6	100 g	20
Special Mix	"	11	"	40
Stewpack Mixed Vegetables	"	6	"	20
Stir Fry Mix	"	14	"	50
Stir Fry Sweetcorn Mix	"	20	"	70
Sweetcorn	"	27	"	95
SAFEWAY (tinned)				
Broad Beans	1 oz	14	100 g	50
Butter Beans	"	17	"	59
Continental Mix	"	10	"	47
Carrots	"	5	"	19
Garden Peas	"	13	"	47
Instant Mashed Potato (dry)	"	75	"	265
Instant Mashes Potato (reconstituted)	"	17	"	60
Jersey Royal Potatoes	"	15	"	53
Marrowfat Peas	"	27	"	95
Mixed Bean Salad in Sauce	"	23	"	82
Mixed Vegetables	"	10	"	37
Petits Pois	"	23	"	82
Processed Peas	"	23	"	80
Ratatouille	"	13	"	46
Red Kidney Beans	"	29	"	101
Sliced Green Beans	"	6	"	23
Whole Button Mushrooms	"	4	"	13

Vegetables & Pulses

Food	Quantities	Calories	Quantities	Calories
(frozen)				
Baby Carrots	1 oz	5	100 g	19
Broad Beans	"	15	"	53
Broccoli Spears	"	9	"	32
Brussels Sprouts	"	12	"	43
Casserole Mixed Bag	"	5	"	17
Cauliflower	"	5	"	19
Chopped Spinach	"	9	"	32
Corn on the Cob	"	36	"	127
Countryside Mixed Veg	"	10	"	36
Courgettes	"	7	"	25
Creamed Spinach	"	11	"	39
Economy Peas	"	15	"	53
Leaf Spinach	"	9	"	31
Minted Peas	"	23	"	82
Mixed Peppers	"	4	"	14
Mixed Vegetables	"	8	"	27
Oriental Stir Fry	"	7	"	26
Oven Chips	"	36	"	125
Peas	"	22	"	78
Petits Pois	"	15	"	53
Potato Chips	"	32	"	112
Rissotto Stir Fry	"	21	"	75
Sliced Green Beans	"	10	"	35
Sliced Onions	"	7	"	23
Southern Stir Fry	"	16	"	55
Special Mixed Veg	"	13	"	45

Food	Quantities	Calories	Quantities	Calories
Sweet Corn	1 oz	36	100 g	127
Whole Green Beans	″	13	″	45

SAINSBURY
Crispy Coated Cauliflower	1 oz	52	100 g	185
Croquettes	″	28	″	98
Jacket Potatoes				
Cottage Cheese & Onion	½ potato	235	″	135
Sweetcorn & Peppers	″	190	″	110
Potatoes, Chipped & Fried	″	35	″	123
Potato Waffles	″	82	″	290
Stir Fried Baby Sweetcorn	″	18	″	65
Stir Fried Mangetouts	″	27	″	95

SPAR (tinned)
Carrots, sliced or whole	1 oz	7	100 g	25
Broad Beans	″	14	″	50
Butter Beans	″	27	″	95
Cut Green Beans	″	18	″	65
Garden Peas	″	13	″	47
Grilling Mushrooms	″	6	″	21
Instant Mashed Potato	″	19	″	66
Marrowfat Processed Peas	″	23	″	81
New Potatoes	″	17	″	60
Processed Peas	″	23	″	81
Red Kidney Beans	″	23	″	82

Vegetables & Pulses

Food	Quantities	Calories	Quantities	Calories
WAITROSE *(tinned)*				
American Red Kidney Beans	1 oz	23	100 g	82
American Sweet Corn	,,	25	,,	90
American Sweetcorn with Peppers	,,	23	,,	82
Asparagus Cuts & Tips	,,	8	,,	27
Asparagus Large Spears	,,	7	,,	25
Baby Carrots	,,	8	,,	29
Butter Beans	,,	27	,,	95
Canadian Green Asparagus	,,	6	,,	21
Celery Hearts	,,	6	,,	15
Chick Peas	,,	21	,,	75
Chopped Mushrooms	,,	6	,,	20
Chopped Spinach	,,	8	,,	30
Cream-Style Corn	,,	23	,,	82
Crushed Tomatoes	,,	6	,,	21
Cut Green Beans	,,	5	,,	19
Garden Peas	,,	13	,,	47
Green Beans, Whole	,,	7	,,	26
Hearts of Artichokes	,,	6	,,	23
Haricots Verts	,,	7	,,	25
Jersey Potatoes	,,	23	,,	80
Macedoine of Vegetables	,,	13	,,	45
Mixed Vegetables	,,	16	,,	58
Passata	,,	6	,,	21
Petits Pois	,,	23	,,	61
Petits Pois & Baby Carrots	,,	18	,,	65

Food	Quantities	Calories	Quantities	Calories
Potatoes	1 oz	18	100 g	64
Processed Peas	,,	27	,,	95
Ratatouille	,,	13	,,	46
Red Kidney Beans in Chilli Sauce	,,	27	,,	95
Saute Potatoes	,,	35	,,	125
with Eggs, Onion & Bacon	,,	48	,,	170
with Onion, Sausages & Cheese	,,	34	,,	120
Sweet Red Peppers	,,	5	,,	18
Swiss Style Potato Fry	,,	38	,,	135
Tomato Puree	,,	24	,,	86
Whole Button Mushrooms *(frozen)*	,,	6	,,	20
Brussels Sprouts	,,	5	,,	18
Broccoli	,,	7	,,	26
Cauliflower Florets	,,	4	,,	13
Corn Cobs	,,	36	,,	127
Garden Peas	,,	15	,,	53
Peas, Mint	,,	15	,,	53
Peas Corn & Pepper	,,	19	,,	68
Petits Pois	,,	15	,,	53
Oven Chips	,,	45	,,	158
Sliced Whole Green Beans	,,	10	,,	35
Stewpack 'Stir Fry'	,,	10	,,	35

Vegetables & Pulses

Food	Quantities	Calories	Quantities	Calories
Cauliflower, Mushrooms Peas	1 oz	12	100 g	44
Courgettes, Corn, Mushrooms	"	16	"	55
Rice, Corn & Prawns	"	33	"	115
Straight Cut Chips	"	32	"	115

Vegetarian Products

This section is new for this edition as there is now a fair selection of tinned, frozen and packaged products on the market suitable for vegetarians. Only those items specifically recommended by the producer for vegetarians are included in this section. There are many more which could probably be eaten in the *Main Meals* and **Vegetable and Pulses** sections but it was thought safer to only include those labelled 'Vegetarian' under this heading. Beware however, because these products can be high in calories.

Food	Quantities	Calories	Quantities	Calories
ALLINSON				
'Vegetable Gourmet'				
Ravioli Verdi	1 serving	264	100 g	132
Vegetable Dhansak	"	114	"	57
Vegetable Sweet & Sour	"	234	"	117
BE-WELL				
Bean Stew Mix	1 oz	98	100 g	349
Haricot Bean Goulash	"	95	"	337
Lentil Curry Mix	"	97	"	344

Vegetarian Products

Food	Quantities	Calories	Quantities	Calories
Spaghetti Bean Bolo	1 oz	98	100 g	348

BOOTS
'Vegetarian Ready Meals'

Food	Quantities	Calories	Quantities	Calories
Country Casserole	1 oz	22	100 g	78
Country Cereal Mix	"	104	"	367
Farmhouse Lentil Mix	"	99	"	349
Harvest Nut Mix	"	116	"	410
Lasagne	"	29	"	103
Ratatouille	"	8	"	30
Risotto	"	38	"	133
TVP Mince	"	93	"	329
TVP Strips	"	93	"	329
Vegetable Burger Mix	"	80	"	281
Vegetable Curry	"	24	"	84
Vegetable Sausage Mix	"	133	"	468

GRANOSE

Food	Quantities	Calories	Quantities	Calories
Bean & Mushroom Stew	1 oz	22	100 g	78
Bologna/Vegelinks	"	47	"	167
Burger Mix	"	128	"	455
Chinese Tofu	"	17	"	60
Curry	"	21	"	76
Curry – Chinese Style	"	16	"	57
Dinner Balls	"	41	"	145
Frikaletts	"	40	"	120
Goulash	"	15	"	54

Food	Quantities	Calories	Quantities	Calories
Hazelnut Paté	1 oz	39	100 g	140
Lentil Roast	”	95	”	336
Lentil & Veg. Casserole	”	28	”	100
Meatless Savoury Cuts	”	25	”	88
Mexican Bean Stew	”	37	”	130
Mexican Corn Roast	”	124	”	440
Nutbrawn	”	60	”	212
Nut Loaf	”	50	”	176
Nut Roast	”	138	”	488
Nuttolene	”	84	”	298
Protose	”	45	”	158
Ravioli	”	18	”	63
Sausalatas	”	39	”	137
Sausfry	”	139	”	492
Saviand	”	56	”	198
Savoury Pudding	”	58	”	207
Savoury Pudding, Country Style	”	47	”	167
Soya Franks	”	85	”	300
Soyapro Beef	”	59	”	210
Chicken	”	59	”	210
Wieners	”	59	”	210
Soya Wurst – Chicken Flavour	”	128	”	455
Tender Bits	”	22	”	79
Tofu in Savoury Bean Sauce	”	34	”	120

Vegetarian Products

Food	Quantities	Calories	Quantities	Calories
Tofu in Tomato Sauce	1 oz	25	100 g	90
HERA				
Bran Rissole	33 g (dry)	108	100 g	324
Complete Pizza Mix	”	266	”	332
Complete Samosas Mix	”	193	”	344
Couscous with Veg. Kofte	76 g (dry)	281	”	370
Fibre-Rich Burgers	33 g (dry)	114	”	339
Savoury Risotta Mix	66 g	228	”	345
Vegetable				
Bolognese	33 g	110	”	333
Casserole	”	116	”	351
Cottage Pie	71 g	278	”	391
Curry	33 g	115	”	348
Goulash	”	117	”	352
Loaf Mix	38 g	166	”	483
Meatballs	33 g	123	”	369
Soysage	”	136	”	408
Stew with Dumplings	56 g	192	”	343
Stroganov	33 g	122	”	367
Supreme	50 g	190	”	380
HOLLAND & BARRETT				
Lentil Dahl	1 oz	30	100 g	105
Mexican Style				
Red Kidney Beans	”	25	”	90
Mixed Bean Salad	”	19	”	67

Food	Quantities	Calories	Quantities	Calories
'Soya Protein' (hydrated)				
Chunks	1 oz	27	100 g	97
Mince	"	27	"	97
Savoury Chunks	"	31	"	110
Savoury Mince	"	31	"	110
Vegetable Curry	"	23	"	83
Vindaloo Curry	"	23	"	82
HOLLY MILLS *(Mixes)*				
'Vegetarian Mixes'				
English	60 g pack	157	100 g	262
Hungarian	"	168	"	280
Italian	"	162	"	270
Mexican	"	157	"	262
Savoury Rissole	184 g pack	602	"	327
MARKS & SPENCER				
Vegetable				
Bake	1 oz	33	100 g	118
Chilli	"	27	"	95
Cutlets	"	30	"	106
Lasagne	"	25	"	87
Samosa	"	69	"	242
MR FRITZIFRY'S				
Hawaiin Croquettes	1 oz	106	100 g	374
Savoury Mix	"	135	"	474

Vegetarian Products

Food	Quantities	Calories	Quantities	Calories
Soy Sausage Mix	1 oz	151	100 g	533
PREWETT'S				
'Just For One' Meals (dry)				
Neapolitan Veg & Spaghetti	1 serving	334	100 g	304
Savoury Veg & Spaghetti	"	339	"	308
Vegetable Curry & Rice	"	331	"	301
'Main Course' (dry)				
Brazilian Style	1 oz	110	100 g	388
Bacon Flavour	"	106	"	373
Beef Flavour	"	106	"	374
Chicken Flavour	"	106	"	374
Sausage/Herbs	"	105	"	372
Savoury Rissole	"	106	"	376
'Ready Meals' (tinned)				
Bolognese Sauce	1 serving	86	"	43
Cannelloni	"	206	"	103
Lasagne	"	182	"	91
Lentil Stew	"	138	"	69
Ravioli	"	166	"	83
Tortellini	"	166	"	83
Vegetable Curry	"	150	"	75
PROTOVEG MENU				
Burgamix	1 oz	153	100 g	539
Farmhouse Soya Stew	"	102	"	357
Jumbo Grills	"	94	"	241

Food	Quantities	Calories	Quantities	Calories
Minced Soya & Onion Mix	1 oz	102	100 g	358
Sizzles	"	159	"	561
Soya Bolognese	"	97	"	343
Soya Mince with veg.	"	98	"	346
Sosmix	"	148	"	520
Veg. Curry	"	102	"	358
Veg. Goulash	"	100	"	351
SAINSBURY				
Ratatouille	½ pack	65	100 g	35
Vegetable Chilli with				
Cracked Wheat	1 pack	380	"	110
Vegetable Mornay	½ pack	230	"	100
TOFEATA *(dry)*				
Tofu	1 serving	20	100 g	79
Tofu Burgers				
Okara Patties	"	234	"	275
Savoury Burgers	"	355	"	315
Spicy Burgers	"	318	"	282
VECON				
Vegetarian Stock *(dry)*	1 oz	44	100 g	155